LOSE WEIGHT
FAST

DIET JOURNAL

INCLUDES
210
Daily Tips for
Weight Loss!

By Alex A. Lluch,
Health and Fitness Expert and
Author of Over 3 Million Books Sold

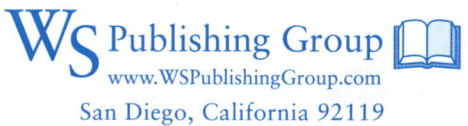
WS Publishing Group
www.WSPublishingGroup.com
San Diego, California 92119

LOSE WEIGHT *FAST* DIET JOURNAL

BY ALEX A. LLUCH

Nutritional and fitness guidelines based on information provided by the United States Food and Drug Administration, Food and Nutrition Information Center, National Agricultural Library, Agricultural Research Service, and the U.S. Department of Agriculture.

Designed by: David Defenbaugh, WS Publishing Group

ISBN-13: 978-1-936061-09-9

Printed in China

DISCLAIMER: The content in this book is provided for general informational purposes only and is not meant to substitute the advice provided by a medical professional. This information is not intended to diagnose or treat medical problems or substitute for appropriate medical care. If you are under the care of a physician and/or take medications for diabetes, heart disease, hypertension, or any other condition, consult your health care provider prior to initiation of any dietary program. Implementation of a dietary program may require altercation in your medication needs and must be done by or under the direction of your physician. If you have or suspect that you have a medical problem, promptly contact your health care provider. Never disregard professional medical advice or delay in seeking it because of something you have read in this book.

Wedding Solutions Publishing, Inc. makes no claims whatsoever regarding the interpretation or utilization of any information contained herein and/or recorded by the user of this journal. If you utilize any information provided in this book, you do so at your own risk and you specifically waive any right to make any claim against the author and publisher, its officers, directors, employees or representatives as the result of the use of such information. Consult your physician before making any changes in your diet or exercise.

TABLE OF CONTENTS

INTRODUCTION **5**

HOW TO USE THIS JOURNAL **7**

YOUR WEIGHT & HEALTH STATUS **11**
- Body Mass Index - BMI 11
- Health Risks and Your Weight 13

SECRETS FOR WEIGHT LOSS **15**
- Suggested Daily Calories for Weight Maintenance 15
- Suggested Daily Calories for Weight Loss 15
- Food Groups, Recommended Daily Amounts 16
- The Nutrition Facts Label 17
- Dietary Guidelines for Americans 18
- Exercise to Jumpstart Weight Loss 19
- Creating a Physical Fitness Program 20
- Revamp Your Daily Routine to Include Fitness 21
- Health Benefits of Physical Activity 22
- Exercise & Weight Control 22
- Calories Burned for Typical Physical Activities 24

YOUR PERSONAL PROFILE **27**
- Your Health Profile 28
- Questions to Ask 30
- Your Goals 31

USING THE JOURNAL PAGES 33

- Daily Journal Pages 33
- Sample Daily Journal Page 35
- Weekly Progress Pages 36
- Sample Weekly Progress Page 37
- Monthly Progress Pages 38
- Sample Monthly Progress Page 40

JOURNAL PAGES 43

- Month 1 84
- Month 2 126
- Month 3 168
- Month 4 210
- Month 5 252
- Month 6 294

NUTRITION FACTS 297

INTRODUCTION

BY PURCHASING THIS BOOK, you have taken the first step in your weight-loss journey to looking and feeling great. Whether you are a veteran of the diet game, or simply want a comprehensive weight-loss program, this is the right book for you!

More than half of American adults today are overweight, with one-third considered obese. America's weight problem has become a serious issue because of the increasing number of diseases linked to being overweight, such as high cholesterol, high blood pressure, diabetes, stroke, and heart disease. We are a nation whose waistline is expanding and will continue to grow unless we take control of our eating habits.

It is difficult in today's society to make the right choices regarding your health and diet. Food portions in restaurants are larger, which encourages us to eat more; our jobs promote sedentary lifestyles; and fast food, while often unhealthy, is convenient and inexpensive. It then becomes the consumer's responsibility to monitor how much he or she eats and to know how much is personally enough. That is where this journal comes in. This journal will facilitate your weight loss in the following ways:

Awareness: Keeping a diet journal builds your daily food awareness. Instead of mindlessly consuming meals, this diet journal will help you become conscious of what you are eating, how much you are eating, and how often you are eating it. This awareness will help you realize that maybe you don't need as much food as you are currently eating. Perhaps you can be perfectly satisfied with less. Once you are aware of what your body needs to lose weight, you can make better, more informed food choices.

Reality: Many dieters do not realize how many calories are included in the foods that they consume. This diet journal allows you to break down your meals into total calories. Then you can see if you have stayed within the range of calories suggested for your diet. For example, if you have a turkey and swiss bagel with mayo, a bag of chips, a chocolate chip cookie, and a soda for lunch, the calories versus a turkey pita with veggies, popcorn, and yogurt would be twice as much. Note the caloric values for both meals:

TURKEY & SWISS BAGEL LUNCH:

370.....large gourmet deli bagel
90 ......3 oz. turkey breast
220 ....2 oz. of swiss cheese
100.....1 tbsp mayo
275.....deli chocolate chip cookie
150.....1 oz. snack bag chips
150.....12 oz. can soda

1,355 .. Total Calories (approx.)

TURKEY PITA LUNCH:

170...whole wheat pita
90 ....3 oz. turkey breast
25 ....1 tbsp grated parmesan cheese
5.......1 tsp mustard
20 ....veggies
60 ....2 cups light microwave popcorn
120 ..6 oz. nonfat flavored yogurt
0.......water with lemon

490...Total Calories (approx.)

Once you realize where your calories are coming from, you can make healthier, low-calorie changes and eliminate the excess foods that do not have significant nutritional value.

Accountability: Keeping a diet journal forces you to account for all food and beverages consumed on a daily basis. When you write down everything you eat and drink, you hold yourself accountable for your intake and see where you might cut back. By calculating the daily nutritional value for all your meals, you can easily see how an extra serving of pasta or a dessert factor into your diet.

Routine: When you start a diet journal, you establish a routine. If you have a plan that you can count on for every day of the week, you are more likely to keep with your diet and avoid situations that can sabotage your diet. By using this diet journal, you are taking charge of your weight-loss program. With this journal as your companion, you can make better, more informed choices that will help you lose weight, look better, and improve your health. Congratulations!

How to Use This Journal

Each section of this diet journal is specifically designed to help guide you through the various stages of your weight-loss program. It will allow you to assess your current health and identify eating behaviors and patterns that may prevent you from losing weight. It provides nutritional guidelines and helps you create realistic goals and expectations as you go through your journey to look better and feel healthier.

YOUR WEIGHT & HEALTH STATUS

Before you begin your keeping your diet journal you should calculate your current status in height, weight, and Body Mass Index (BMI), and assess your health risks based on your waist size.

SECRETS FOR WEIGHT LOSS

Any successful weight-loss program should include an understanding of nutritional guidelines. Nutrition is a multi-faceted concept that includes a wide range of elements. Maintain your program armed with information on the suggested daily calorie intake for weight maintenance/weight loss, USDA Food Guide, the nutrition facts label, and the best sources for essential nutrients.

Additionally, you can use the Calories Burned for Typical Physical Activities table in this chapter to determine how many calories you are burning through various activities you enjoy. Physical activity is a great way to expedite a successful weight-loss program.

YOUR PERSONAL PROFILE

Fill out your personal health profile at the start of your diet so you can accurately assess your current physical state, habits, and eating patterns. Documenting this information will assist you in identifying the areas of your diet and health that need improvement and help you see your personal statistics prior to beginning your diet plan.

You will also include a "Before" photo in this section. You will be amazed at how far you've come as you keep track of your weight-loss progress, reduced body fat percentage, and new measurements in the journal pages.

You will also solidify your weight-loss goals and plans and the means by which you will achieve them. You can map out your target daily intake for calories, fat, carbs, protein and fiber, as well as the physical fitness component you would like to include in your diet plan.

USING THE JOURNAL PAGES

The journal pages are the heart of your program. They are a source of personal feedback and a daily reminder of all the elements of your weight-loss plan. Your daily journal will help you stay focused on your personal goals and reassess your eating habits. These pages will help you keep track of your food and beverage intake, make sure you are within your daily calorie allotment, and ensure that you are getting enough fluids. You will also be able to log your daily weight, vitamins and supplements, energy levels, servings, and calories burned. At the end of each week and each month, you can record your weight loss and evaluate whether or not you were able to meet the goals you set for that time period.

YOUR WEIGHT-LOSS PROGRESS CHART

Use the 6-month fold-out progress chart to track your daily, weekly and monthly progress. Customize the chart according to your personal weight-loss goals. Begin with your starting weight; then, the horizontal lines of the graph signify pounds of weight. Decide how many pounds each horizontal line should represent. For example, if you have a lot of weight to lose, you will probably want each horizontal line to indicate one pound. For moderate weight loss, use every other line to record each pound. The vertical lines indicate days of the week. Each day, place a dot on the line that represents your weight. At the end of the week, write your weight in the bubble at the top of the graph. To chart your progress, simply connect the dots. This is a great way to see a graph of your weight-loss journey over 30 weeks. In addition, this chart includes space to record your end weight, goal and notes for each month.

NUTRITION FACTS

This section is an invaluable resource for determining the right foods for your diet. In this section, look up the calories and nutritional content for fat, protein, carbohydrates, and fiber for more than 1,000 popular food items. Write the corresponding information in your journal to track your daily intake.

GOALS ACHIEVED STICKERS

Place a sticker on each day, weekly progress page or monthly progress page where you have successfully met a goal for that time period.

LOSE WEIGHT FAST DIET JOURNAL TO-GO

This mini journal provides an easy way to stick with your diet plan, even while you're on the go. Take the mini journal with you in a purse, pocket or bag and write down everything you eat and drink, physical activities, energy levels, and notes so you can update the main journal later.

YOUR WEIGHT & HEALTH STATUS

The most important reasons to start a weight-loss program are to look and feel great, and to reduce the risk of health complications such as heart disease and diabetes. Before you start, however, it is important to assess your health status. There are three methods to determine your overall physical condition: your height and weight measurements, waist size, and Body Mass Index (BMI). Another consideration is your family history.

For adults 18 years and older, the first step is to measure your height and weight. Use those two numbers to find your BMI on the following page. If your BMI falls within the range of 19 to 24, you are considered healthy. If your BMI lands from 25 to 29, then you have an increased risk of developing health problems. If your BMI is 30 or above, you could be considered obese. If you fall into the last two categories, it is essential to plan and manage your weight-loss program.

The second factor in evaluating your weight is your waist size. Use a tape measure to calculate your waist circumference below your rib cage and above your belly button. You have an increased health risk for developing serious chronic illness if your waist size is more than 35 inches for women and 40 inches for men.

BODY MASS INDEX - BMI

Body composition can vary greatly from individual to individual. Two people who possess the same height and weight can have different bone structure and varying percentages of muscle and fat. Therefore, your weight alone is not the only factor in assessing your risk for weight-related health issues. Your BMI can help indicate whether or not your health is at risk.

Calculating your BMI: Locate your height in the left-hand column below. Then move across the row to your weight. The number at the very top of the column is your BMI.

BMI	19	20	21	22	23	24	25	26	27	28	29	30	31	32	33	34	35
Height							**Weight in pounds**										
4'10"	91	96	100	105	110	115	119	124	129	134	138	143	148	153	158	162	167
4'11"	94	99	104	109	114	119	124	128	133	138	143	148	153	158	163	168	173
5'	97	102	107	112	118	123	128	133	138	143	148	153	158	163	158	174	179
5'1"	100	106	111	116	122	127	132	137	143	148	153	158	164	169	174	180	185
5'2"	104	109	115	120	126	131	136	142	147	153	158	164	169	175	180	186	191
5'3"	107	113	118	124	130	135	141	146	152	158	163	169	175	180	186	191	197
5'4"	110	116	122	128	134	140	145	151	157	163	169	174	180	186	192	197	204
5'5"	114	120	126	132	(138)	144	150	156	162	168	174	180	186	192	198	204	210
5'6"	118	124	130	136	142	148	155	161	167	173	179	186	192	198	204	210	216
5'7"	121	127	134	140	146	153	159	166	172	178	185	191	198	204	211	217	223
5'8"	125	131	138	144	151	158	164	171	177	184	190	197	203	210	216	223	230
5'9"	128	135	142	149	155	162	169	176	182	189	196	203	209	216	223	230	236
5'10"	132	139	146	153	160	167	174	181	188	195	202	209	216	222	229	236	243
5'11"	136	143	150	157	165	172	179	186	193	200	208	215	222	229	236	243	250
6'	140	147	154	162	169	177	184	191	199	206	213	221	228	235	242	250	258
6'1"	144	151	159	166	174	182	189	197	204	212	219	227	235	242	250	257	265
6'2"	148	155	163	171	179	186	194	202	210	218	225	233	241	249	256	264	272
6'3"	152	160	168	176	184	192	200	208	216	224	232	240	248	256	264	272	279
	Healthy					**Overweight**						**Obese**					

HEALTH RISKS AND YOUR WEIGHT

For most adults, BMI and waist size are fairly reliable indicators of whether or not you are overweight. These two indicators are also effective in assessing your risk of weight-related health issues.

Your waist measurement determines whether or not you have the tendency to carry fat around your midsection. A higher waist size may indicate a greater risk for weight-related health issues such as high blood pressure, type-2 diabetes and coronary artery disease. Typically, the higher your Body Mass Index, the greater risk to your health. This risk also increases if your waist is greater than 35 inches for women or 40 inches for men.

If your weight indicates that you are at a higher risk for health problems, consult your primary care physician to determine safe and effective ways to improve your health. Even moderate amounts of weight loss, around 5 to 10 percent of your weight, can have long-lasting health benefits.

Risk of Associated Disease According to BMI and Waist Size

Body Mass Index		Waist less than or equal to 40" Men 35" Women	Waist greater than 40" Men 35" Women
18 or less	Underweight	N/A	N/A
19-24	Normal	N/A	N/A
25-29	Overweight	Increased	High
30-35	Obese	High	Very High
over 35	Obese	Very High	Very High

SECRETS FOR WEIGHT LOSS

SUGGESTED DAILY CALORIES FOR WEIGHT MAINTENANCE

Your total daily calories should be based on your age, gender, body type, and level of physical activity. Active men should consume approximately 2,800 calories per day to maintain their ideal weight. Active women and sedentary men should eat 2,200 calories. Sedentary women and older adults should strive for 1,600 calories. If you are not sure of how many daily calories you should consume, consult your primary care physician for a recommendation.

1,600 CALORIES	Sedentary women and older adults should consume approximately 1,600 calories daily.
2,200 CALORIES	Most children, teenage girls, active women and sedentary men should consume approximately 2,200 calories daily. Pregnant or breast-feeding women may need to consume more.
2,800 CALORIES	Most teenage boys and active men and some very active women should consume approximately 2,800 calories daily.

SUGGESTED DAILY CALORIES FOR WEIGHT LOSS

The total number of daily calories for a weight-loss plan will depend on the number of pounds you wish to lose. Once you have determined the daily number of calories that you should eat to maintain your weight (based on the chart above), you should decrease your total caloric intake by an average of 500 calories per day for a moderate weight loss. To proceed in a safe and healthy manner, you can eliminate those 500 calories simply by decreasing the amount of sugars, refined carbohydrates, and alcohol in your diet, most of which provide calories with little nutritional value.

FOOD GROUPS, RECOMMENDED DAILY AMOUNTS

The United States Department of Agriculture is known for its Food Guide, which is a nutritional reference for many health groups and dietary plans. The USDA Food Guide separates the foods you should eat into six different categories: 1) grains, 2) vegetables, 3) fruits, 4) fats and oils, 5) milk and dairy products, and 6) meat, beans, fish, and nuts. The suggested amounts below have been developed to help you select the proper amount of food to eat from each group on a daily basis. Each group provides you with a different set of essential nutrients. By following the recommended serving sizes, you can be assured that you are getting the proper amounts of protein, fats, carbohydrates, fiber, vitamins, and minerals. This guide can be adjusted to suit your personal needs.

DAILY AMOUNT OF FOOD FROM EACH GROUP

Daily Calorie Level	1,200	1,400	1,600	1,800	2,000	2,200	2,400	2,600	2,800	3,000
Fruits	1 C (2 srv)	1.5 C (3 srv)	1.5 C (3 srv)	1.5 C (3 srv)	2 C (4 srv)	2 C (4 srv)	2 C (4 srv)	2 C (4 srv)	2.5 C (5 srv)	2.5 C (5 srv)
Vegetables	1.5 C (3 srv)	1.5 C (2 srv)	2 C (4 srv)	2.5 C (5 srv)	2.5 C (5 srv)	3 C (6 srv)	3 C (6 srv)	3.5 C (7 srv)	3.5 C (7 srv)	4 C (8 srv)
Grains	4 oz.	5 oz.	5 oz.	6 oz.	6 oz.	7 oz.	8 oz	9 oz.	10 oz.	10 oz.
Meat, Beans, Fish & Nuts	3 oz.	4 oz.	5 oz.	5 oz.	5.5 oz.	6 oz.	6.5 oz.	6.5 oz.	7 oz.	7 oz
Milk	2 C	2 C	3 C	3 C	3 C	3 C	3 C	3 C	3 C	3 C
Fats & Oils	17 g	17 g	22 g	24 g	27 g	29 g	31 g	34 g	36 g	44 g

Food Group	Food group amounts shown in cups (C) or ounces (oz.), with number of servings (srv) in parentheses. Oils are shown in grams.

THE NUTRITION FACTS LABEL

Most packaged foods have a nutrition facts label. Use this information to make healthy choices quickly and easily.

Nutrition Facts

Serving Size 1 cup (228g)
Servings Per Container 2

Amount per Serving

Calories 250	Calories from Fat 110

% Daily Value*

Total Fat 12g	18%
Saturated Fat 3g	15%
Trans Fat 3g	
Cholesterol 30mg	10%
Sodium 470mg	20%
Total Carbohydrate 31g	10%
Dietary Fiber 0g	0%
Sugars 5g	
Protein 5g	

Vitamin A	4%
Vitamin C	2%
Calcium	20%
Iron	4%

* Percent Daily Values are based on a 2,000 calorie diet. Your Daily Values may be higher or lower depending on your calorie needs.

	Calories:	2,000	2,500
Total Fat	Less than	65g	80g
Sat Fat	Less than	20g	25g
Cholesterol	Less than	300mg	300mg
Sodium	Less than	2,400mg	2,400mg
Total Carbohydrate		300g	375g
Dietary Fiber		25g	30g

LABEL AT A GLANCE

Start Here: Check the serving size and servings per container.

Calories: 400 or more calories per serving is considered high. Note the calories from fat.

Daily Values: 5%=low, 20%=high.

Limit These Nutrients: Eating too much fat, saturated fat, trans fat, cholesterol, or sodium may put you at an increased health risk for diseases such as heart disease, some cancers, or high blood pressure.

Get Enough of These Nutrients: Most Americans do not receive the proper amount of fiber, vitamins A and C, calcium or iron from their diets. Eating enough of these nutrients can limit your risk of diseases such as osteoporosis and heart disease.

Daily Values Footnote: This footnote makes recommendations for key nutrients based on diets of 2,000 and 2,500 daily calories.

DIETARY GUIDELINES FOR AMERICANS

1. Including various foods in your diet will allow your body to receive the energy (calories), protein, vitamins, minerals, and fiber you need to maintain proper health.

2. Combine a healthy diet with physical activity to improve your weight or maintain your weight. Maintaining a healthy weight reduces the risk of related diseases, such as high blood pressure, heart disease, a stroke, certain cancers, and the most common kind of diabetes.

3. Choose a diet low in fat, saturated fat and cholesterol to reduce your risk of heart disease and certain types of cancer. Because fat contains more than twice the calories of an equal amount of carbohydrates or protein, a diet low in fat can help you maintain a healthy weight.

4. Include plenty of vegetables, fruits, and whole grain products in your diet. These foods provide essential vitamins, minerals, fiber, and complex carbohydrates. They are also generally lower in fat.

5. Use sugars only in moderation. A diet with high amounts of sugars has unnecessary calories and too few nutrients for the majority of adults. Excess sugar can also contribute to tooth decay.

6. Use salt and other forms of sodium in moderation to help reduce your risk of high blood pressure.

7. If you drink alcoholic beverages, do so in moderation. Alcoholic beverages supply calories, but little or no nutrients. Drinking alcohol is also the cause of many health problems and accidents and can lead to addiction.

EXERCISE TO JUMPSTART WEIGHT LOSS

A key element for weight-loss success is developing an exercise program. Choose activities that can be done each day so you can incorporate them into your daily routine. The length of time it takes to change from a sedentary to an active lifestyle can range from three weeks to three months. Get started by creating simple habits like taking walking more often when you're going somewhere in your neighborhood. Slowly add more exercises and increase the intensity as your body adjusts to each new activity.

So what is the best exercise regiment for you to embark on? The answer depends on your personality, interests, and individual abilities. The optimal solution is to choose an exercise program you will enjoy doing, and one that you will look forward to each day.

You have a wide range of options when creating a fitness plan. It can be slow, moderate, or physically challenging. You can do it all at one time, or integrate it into two or three segments over the course of your day. So build a physical activity plan that fits into your daily calendar, and keep in mind the common ingredient for any successful exercise program is to bring a measure of pleasure into it.

In addition to having fun and feeling energized, you will find that physical activity provides added perks, such as building muscle tone, curbing your appetite, and increasing your metabolism. One by-product built into a fitness-oriented lifestyle is improved overall health. It has been found that regular physical exercise reduces the risks of cancer, cardiovascular disease, and diabetes. It also provides psychological benefits, such as increased self-esteem and feelings of confidence. Getting more physically fit will have you feeling strong, mentally and physically, and will make you look great, too.

CREATING A PHYSICAL FITNESS PROGRAM

Your mission is to burn calories. Your new fitness program should include three essential elements for successful, long-term weight loss and maintenance: the first element is to include aerobic activities, which provide cardiovascular benefits; the second element is a resistance or strength-training program for improving muscle tone; and the third element is to consider integrating a basic stretching routine into your daily schedule to develop flexibility.

Before embarking on your mission, see a doctor to obtain a health clearance if you have unique health issues, injuries, or physical limitations. When you are ready to exercise, warm up slowly and be gentle on your body. It's the only one you've got, so take care of it as you work your way into top physical form.

Aerobic Activities: An aerobic activity is any type of body movement that speeds up your heart rate and breathing. It improves your ability to utilize oxygen, which increases your cardiovascular health. You can participate in aerobic activities almost anywhere: taking step classes at a gym, running in a park or riding a stationary bicycle in your home environment. The minimum amount of time for adult daily exercise is 30 minutes, and children benefit from 60 minutes per day. Keep in mind these numbers are a general estimate and should be tailored to fit individual needs. In all cases, use common sense when exercising and be sure to listen to your body. A general guideline for physical activity is to safely challenge your body while gradually stretching your limits.

Resistance & Strength Training: Once you have a personalized aerobic program that fits your style, consider adding a crucial piece of the puzzle to your fitness regime. Resistance and strength training will firm up muscles as the unwanted pounds melt away. This type of exercise should be done for 20 to 30 minutes, three times a week. It includes lifting handheld weights, using machines at a gym, or working out with videos in your home. If you choose to go to the gym, consult with professionals and learn how to correctly use the equipment.

Stretching & Flexibility: Stretching and flexibility are often neglected components of physical activity. Preparing the body for movement and keeping it injury-free should be built into every fitness program. Stretching and flexibility training is designed to develop range of motion, increase muscle elasticity, and achieve muscle balance. Stretching can also speed up recovery in preparation for the next fitness session. You should never stretch your body when it's cold or stiff. Be sure to start your physical activity with 10 to 15 minutes of slow movement until your muscles have warmed up. Mild stretching can be done at a midpoint in your daily training and again at the completion of the exercise program.

The best type of overall stretching routine is one that starts with the head and neck, working down toward the toes. It uses slow stretches that are held for a minimum of 10 seconds each. Avoid quick-pulling motions that put stress on muscles and joints. Choose abdominal exercises that support the lower back region. In all cases, consult with a professional for advice before beginning a strength and flexibility program.

REVAMP YOUR DAILY ROUTINE TO INCLUDE FITNESS

If you are not the type of person who enjoys going to a gym, consider making your home environment a personalized recreational center. All forms of physical activity burn calories. So let's look at your daily chores in a new light: vacuuming for one hour burns 220 calories, grocery shopping requires 180 calories, and raking leaves expends 90 calories. If you have access to stairs, perhaps you might use them as your personal stair stepper. Walking up stairs in an easy and moderate manner for 15 minutes burns 120 calories.

Enjoy being outdoors? Try an afternoon of gardening, sweeping, raking leaves or mowing the lawn to tone up your arms, legs, and abs while you whittle away an additional 270 calories per hour. If you live in an area where it snows, you have hit the jackpot as shoveling snow consumes almost 600 calories per hour. Combining a few of these forms of aerobic activity is the equivalent of spending a couple of hours in the gym.

HEALTH BENEFITS OF PHYSICAL ACTIVITY

Still need convincing that it is essential to change from a sedentary lifestyle to one that includes daily physical activity? Here are a few facts that might influence your decision: it has been found that regular physical activity reduces the risk of dying prematurely; exercise reduces the risk of developing heart disease, cancer, diabetes, and high blood pressure, and promotes psychological well-being. Exercise also helps decrease or eliminate depression and anxiety. Participating in physical activities is also an effective way to lose weight and maintain weight loss.

EXERCISE & WEIGHT CONTROL

Did you know that being overweight and being "overfat" are two different dilemmas? Some people, such as athletes, have a muscular physique and weigh more than average for their age and height. But their body composition, which is the amount of fat versus lean body mass (muscle, bone, organs and tissue), is within an acceptable range. Others can weigh within the range of U.S. guidelines, yet they can carry around too much fat. Use exercise as a way to balance your body fat percentage. An easy self-test is to pinch the thickness of fat at your waist and abdomen. If you can pinch more than an inch of fat, excluding muscles, chances are you have too much body fat.

Carrying around too much body fat is a pain. Many people fight the battle of the bulge through diet alone because exercise is not always convenient. Many people spend hours behind desks and computers. In addition, much of our leisure time is spent in sedentary pursuits. To reverse this trend, it is important to adjust your attitude and find time to exercise each day.

Common excuses people use to avoid physical activity include:

1. "I don't have the time."
2. "I'm too tired and I don't feel like it."

3. "I'm not very good at exercising."
4. "It's not convenient to get to my workout place."
5. "I'm afraid and embarrassed."
6. "It's too expensive to join a gym."

Write down the reasons you've been avoiding exercise, joining a gym, or taking a fitness class. Now write down solutions to these reasons, which are really just excuses. For example, if your number one reason for skipping exercise is "I don't have time," you might consider taking half your lunch break to go for a walk or going for a bike ride with your family instead of going out for dinner.

FITNESS SOLUTIONS

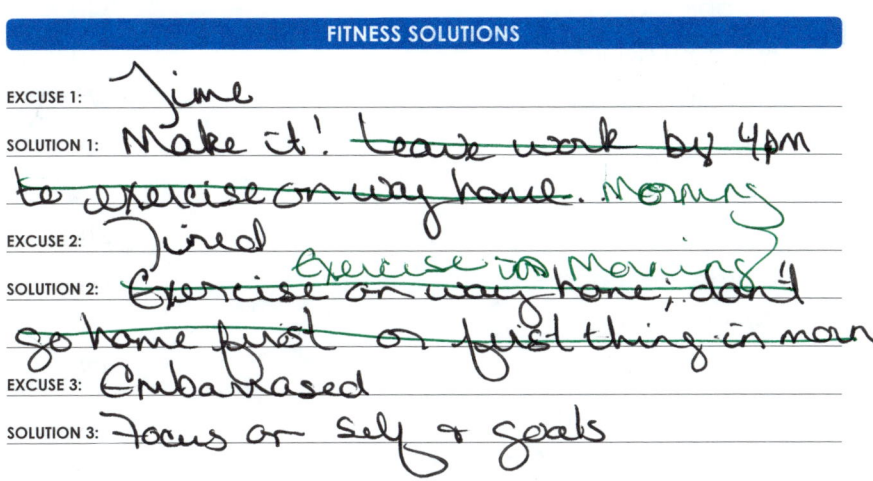

EXCUSE 1: *Time*

SOLUTION 1: *Make it! Leave work by 4pm to exercise on way home. Morning*

EXCUSE 2: *Tired*

SOLUTION 2: *Exercise on way home, don't go home first or first thing in morn.*

EXCUSE 3: *Embarrased*

SOLUTION 3: *Focus on self & goals*

There is never a good excuse to be sedentary. There are great gyms and fitness facilities of all types and price ranges. If you find the traditional gym environment isn't for you, try taking up a yoga or dance class. If money is a concern, sign up for a hiking club — things like hiking, swimming, rollerblading and biking are always free. The website MeetUp.com is great for finding groups of people with your similar interests in your area. Flip to the next page, to the Calories Burned for Typical Physical Activities chart, and look at how many ways there are to burn calories!

CALORIES BURNED FOR TYPICAL PHYSICAL ACTIVITIES

Light Activities: 150 or less	Cal/Hr.
Billiards	140
Lying down/sleeping	60
Office work	140
Sitting	80
Standing	100

Moderate Activities: 150-350	Cal/Hr.
Aerobic dancing	340
Ballroom dancing	210
Bicycling (5 mph)	170
Bowling	160
Canoeing (2.5 mph)	170
Dancing (social)	210
Gardening (moderate)	270
Golf (with cart)	180
Golf (without cart)	320
Grocery shopping	180
Horseback riding (sitting trot)	250
Light housework/cleaning, etc.	250
Ping-pong	270
Swimming (20 yards/min)	290
Tennis (recreational doubles)	310
Vacuuming	220
Volleyball (recreational)	260
Walking (2 mph)	200
Walking (3 mph)	240
Walking (4 mph)	300

CALORIES BURNED FOR TYPICAL PHYSICAL ACTIVITIES

Vigorous Activities: 350 or MORE	Cal/Hr.
Aerobics (step)	440
Backpacking (10 lb load)	540
Badminton	450
Basketball (competitive)	660
Basketball (leisure)	390
Bicycling (10 mph)	375
Bicycling (13 mph)	600
Cross country skiing (leisurely)	460
Cross country skiing (moderate)	660
Hiking	460
Ice skating (9 mph)	384
Jogging (5 mph)	550
Jogging (6 mph)	690
Racquetball	620
Rollerblading	384
Rowing machine	540
Running (8 mph)	900
Scuba diving	570
Shoveling snow	580
Soccer	580
Spinning	650
Stair climber machine	480
Swimming (50 yards/min.)	680
Water aerobics	400
Water skiing	480
Weight training (30 sec. btwn sets)	760
Weight training (60 sec. btwn sets)	570

YOUR PERSONAL PROFILE

Begin your weight-loss program by gathering some information to assess your current physical state, habits, and eating patterns. This information will assist you in identifying the areas of your diet and health that need improvement, as well as your progress.

On the following page, fill in your age, weight, height, body fat percentage, and Body Mass Index. Visit your primary care physician and have your cholesterol, triglycerides, and blood pressure measured. This information will help you determine if you are at risk for certain diseases or conditions. These levels will also factor into the food choices you make when creating your diet. For example, if you have high blood pressure, you will want to reduce your sodium intake.

Next, assess your current eating and physical habits. You will also answer some additional questions about your eating habits to help you define problem areas.

You should also place a "Before" photo in this chapter. Take your current measurements. You will be tracking your weight loss and muscle gain throughout this journal. It will be wonderfully motivating to look back and see a visual of where you began and how far you have come throughout your weight-loss journey.

Finally, outline your diet plan and your diet and exercise goals. Record the specific amounts of daily calories, fats, carbs, protein and fiber your plan includes. This will help you stay within your total daily allotments when you are making food choices and filling out the daily journal pages. Use this section to outline the physical activities you would like to include in a fitness plan and schedule them into your week. Good luck meeting all your goals!

YOUR HEALTH PROFILE

Complete the following personal health profile. You can request necessary information from your primary health care provider.

Name: _____   Triglycerides: _____

Age: _42_____   HDL Cholesterol: _____

Height: _5'5_____   LDL Cholesterol: _____

Total cholesterol: _____   Blood Pressure: _____

Current Diet & Eating Habits: (fast food, snack often, late-night eating, etc.)

fast food ; bored eating ; grazing
_____
_____

Current Physical Activity: (sedentary, moderately active, very active)

sedentary ; very active on occasion
_____
_____

Other Current Habits: (smoking, drinking, lack of sleep, etc.)

lack of sleep; working late into night
_____
_____

DATE:_____   WEIGHT:_____   BODY FAT %:_____

MEASUREMENTS:

____ chest   ____ biceps   ____ waist   ____ hips   ____ thighs

COMMENTS:_____

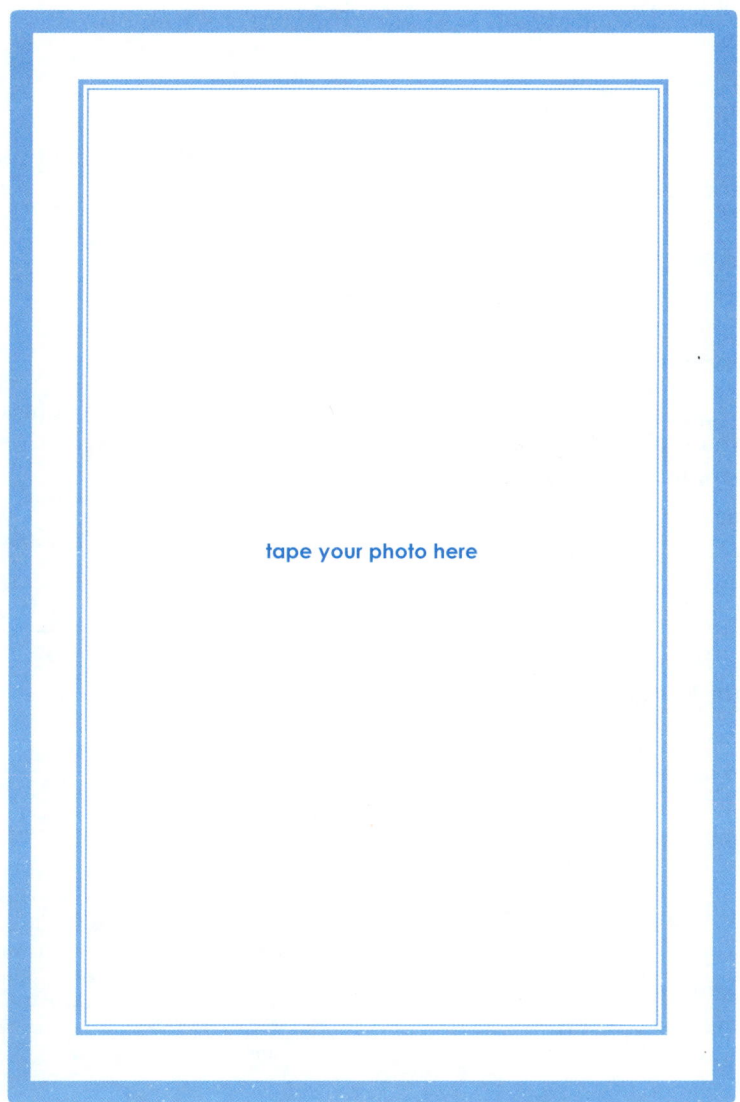

tape your photo here

The following questions will assist you in developing your weight-loss program. When choosing a specific diet program, determining your strengths and weaknesses will help you figure out what plan is right for you.

QUESTIONS TO ASK

Which best describes your daily eating habits?

- ☐ Three average meals
- ☑ Graze frequently
- ☑ One large meal and little else

What types of food do you crave the most?

- ☐ Meat/fish
- ☐ Fruit/vegetables
- ☑ Bread/cereals/rice
- ☐ Sweets

Do you typically eat out or prepare food for yourself?

- ☐ I usually cook my own food
- ☑ I eat out or have premade meals

What is your weight-loss goal?

- ☑ Lose 20 or more pounds
- ☐ Maintain weight
- ☐ Lose a little weight
- ☑ Improve health

What is your fitness goal?

- ☑ Decrease fat
- ☐ Gain muscle
- ☑ Improve strength

Describe your body type:

- ☑ Overweight
- ☐ Average
- ☐ Muscular

What length of plan would you like to have?

- ☐ Less than 1 month
- ☐ 1-3 months
- ☑ 3-6 months
- ☐ 6 or more months

For what particular event (if any) do you want to lose weight?

_____

_____

_____

_____

_____

NOTE:

When developing your weight-loss program and goals, be sure to take into account the answers that you have noted above. These answers will factor into your decision when choosing the program that would be most effective and best suited to your needs.

Complete the following information based on your diet and intake goals:

YOUR GOALS

YOUR DIET GOALS	2 2 7 #

(handwritten notes, mostly crossed out)

- 10% by Aug 15 / / 123 lbs
- 20% by Dec 1 / / ~ 40 lbs
- remainder by Feb 1 / / 18 lbs

10# per mth   — 180 by July

YOUR INTAKE GOALS

Based on the number of calories your diet allows, list the daily targets that you would like to meet. (Your primary care physician can help you determine the appropriate amounts.)

DAILY CALORIES:	FAT gms:	CARBS gms:	PROTEIN gms:	FIBER gms:
1600				

NOTES:

Write your goals for physical activity for each day of the week:

YOUR EXERCISE GOALS

MONDAY: TreadClimber 25 mins AM
Walk dog 20 mins PM

TUESDAY:

WEDNESDAY:

THURSDAY:

FRIDAY:

SAT/SUN:

NOTES:

Using the
Journal Pages

These journal pages are the most important part of your weight-loss journey; recording your nutritional intake and other daily factors will help you cut calories, shed pounds, and develop healthy eating habits in the long-run.

Each daily journal page allows you to record as much or as little information as you like. Just remember that the best way to lose weight is to write down every bite and snack you eat, as well as monitor your energy levels, water intake, calories burned and more. Each journal page also includes a daily tip for eating smart, losing weight, and getting fit, which will help inspire and motivate you.

Here is an explanation of the different components of the journal pages:

DAILY JOURNAL PAGES

1 Weight: Document your daily weight on each journal page. Invest in a scale so you can accurately measure your progress. Weigh yourself unclothed when you wake up in the morning, before breakfast, so you can get a fresh reading for the day. Write this number in the space provided. Keep in mind that there are many factors, such as water and muscle gain, that can affect your weight. Don't let a small weight gain thwart your program; instead, focus more on your weekly and monthly progress.

2 Daily Nutritional Intake: Write down all the foods you eat on a daily basis in your journal, including all meals, snacks, sauces, dressings, condiments, and beverages.

For each item, record the quantity and total amount of calories, fat, carbs, protein and fiber. You can find the values for more than 1,000 popular food items in the back of this journal. In addition, you can refer to the Nutritional Facts label printed on the container of most prepackaged foods. Once you have made all of your documentation for the day, use the Daily Totals section to calculate the total amounts you have consumed. Compare your totals to the number of calories suggested for your program. If you are at your target or under, you are on the right track. If you are a little over, don't worry. Just make some adjustments to your diet and try to choose more low-calorie options. Do your best to avoid diet pitfalls, such as sugar, extra fat, and alcohol.

3 **Water Intake:** Strive for a total of eight 8-ounce glasses of water per day. Check off a box for each 8-ounce glass you drink each day. Many times, people believe that they are hungry when they are actually thirsty. If you drink water on a regular basis throughout the day, you can keep your metabolism and bodily functions working at optimum levels.

4 **Energy Level:** Determine the relationship that your body has with food. Take notice of how your body responds to your weight-loss program. Document your daily overall energy by checking one of the three boxes in this section. See how your energy correlates to the types of foods you have eaten that day. For example, if you notice that a little extra protein helps you get through your workout, incorporate lean meats in your diet. As you discover these relationships, make adjustments as needed to help you feel your best.

5 **Daily Number of Servings:** Record the number of servings you get from each of the six major food groups — fruits, vegetables, grains, meats and beans, milk and dairy, and oils and sweets. Refer to the table in the chapter "Secrets for Weight Loss" to determine how many servings you should be getting from each group to maintain a balanced diet plan.

6 **Vitamins & Supplements:** This section is a great daily reminder if you are incorporating additional nutrients into your diet program. If you are restricting your daily caloric intake, it can be a good idea to

TUESDAY

I Did It!
DAILY GOALS ACHIEVED

DAILY NUTRITIONAL INTAKE

Food/Beverages	Qty.	Calories	Fat	Carbs.	Protein	Fiber
Blueberry scone	1	400	17	55	5	2
Orange juice	12 oz.	110	0	26	2	0
Bagel w/turkey		490	4	70	30	3
American cheese	2	64	2	2	8	0
Baby carrots		100	0	24	3	5
Pepsi	12 oz.	180	0	45	0	0
Apple slices and		245	17	21	10	4
peanut butter						
Salmon	8 oz.	416	22	0	68	0
Wild rice		166	2	34	7	3
Broccoli		54	1	12	2	3
Crystal Light tea		5	0	0	0	0
DAILY TOTALS:		2,230	65	289	135	21

2

DAILY EXERCISE

Activity	Hrs./Mins.	Cal. Burned
Yoga	60 mins	300
DAILY TOTALS:		300

7

TIP OF THE DAY!

The gratification of gradual weight loss will be much more satisfying than the instant gratification of food.

8

DAILY NOTES, ACHIEVEMENTS

Obstacles, solutions, and thoughts on your progress.

Need more fiber during breakfast! Buy oatmeal.

Do 30 minutes of cardio tomorrow. **9**

DATE:
06/23

WEIGHT:
197

WATER INTAKE:
# of 8oz. glasses
☑ ☑ ☑ ☑
☑ ☑ ☐ **3**

ENERGY LEVEL:
☐ low **4**
☑ medium
☐ high

DAILY # OF SERVINGS: **5**
3 fruits
2 veggies
3 grains
2 meats & beans
1 milk & dairy
3 oils & sweets

VITAMINS & SUPPLEMENTS:
Calcium **6**
vitamin C

take vitamins and supplements. If you choose to do so, write it in your journal and be sure to keep track on a daily basis. You can also assess the effectiveness of your supplements over time by comparing your energy levels to the vitamins that you have taken. Also, if you make changes to food that you eat while on your diet, you may want to consider adapting your supplements as well. When in doubt about specific vitamin recommendations, consult with a health care professional.

7 Daily Exercise: This section will encourage you to participate in exercise on a daily basis. All physical activity burns calories, so be sure to refer to the "Calories Burned for Typical Physical Activities" section in this book. Since weight loss is determined by the amount of calories consumed versus the amount burned, if you happen to have a "bad eating day" you can make up for the extra calories by adding exercise to that day or another day that week.

8 Tip of the Day!: Use this daily tip as a reminder for ways to eat smart and be healthy, as well as to stay motivated throughout your diet plan.

9 Daily Notes, Achievements: This section will help you observe obstacles and solutions throughout your diet journey. Record your thoughts and feelings as you gradually achieve your weight-loss goals. Stay motivated by recording positive results and reflecting on your progress. If for any reason you did not meet your daily goal, reflect on the factors that kept you from your goal and write them down in this section. You can then decide on any changes to your diet or fitness plan that will help you stay on track. Incorporate these improvements into the following day.

WEEKLY PROGRESS PAGES

Use these journal pages to record your start and end weight, days you tracked your diet, days you exercised, total calories burned for the week, and weekly energy level. The Weekly Progress pages will give you an

WEEKLY PROGRESS

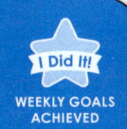

I Did It!
WEEKLY GOALS
ACHIEVED

HIGHLIGHT OF THE WEEK

Your single-greatest moment of the week!

I met my goal from last week to run a mile in under 9 minutes! Pretty cool!

1

START WEIGHT:

197

END WEIGHT:

195

NUTRITIONAL INTAKE WRAP-UP

Did you meet your intake goals for the week? Why or why not?

I went to the movies with friends, and I didn't order a large popcorn like I usually do. I did have a few handfuls of Joe's popcorn. Next time, I'm going to sit next to someone who isn't eating popcorn.

2

DAYS I TRACKED MY DIET:

- ☑ Mon.
- ☑ Tues.
- ☑ Wed.
- ☑ Thurs.
- ☑ Fri.
- ☐ Sat.
- ☑ Sun.

EXERCISE WRAP-UP

Did you meet your exercise goals for the week? Why or why not?

I skipped my workout on Thursday to go to the movies with friends. Next time, I should plan to run in the morning if I have something to do at night.

3

DAYS I EXERCISED:

- ☑ Mon.
- ☑ Tues.
- ☑ Wed.
- ☐ Thurs.
- ☐ Fri.
- ☑ Sat.
- ☐ Sun.

GOALS FOR NEXT WEEK

Things to work on for next week.

I am going to dinner with a friend next Wednesday, and I would like to avoid sharing an appetizer or drinking more than one beer.

I don't want to pass on plans with friends but I don't want to skip any workouts either.

4

WEEKLY CALORIES BURNED:

950

WEEKLY ENERGY LEVEL:

- ☐ low
- ☑ medium
- ☐ high

accurate picture of how you did and how you felt for each week.

1 **Highlight of the Week:** Writing down the highlight of your week as it relates to diet and weight loss can be very motivating and keeps your spirits high. For instance, if you met your goal from the previous week, document that here.

2 **Nutritional Intake Wrap-Up:** At the end of each week, evaluate how well you did at meeting your intake goals. If you met your goals, write down what worked for you. If you went over your allotted intake, describe what kept you from meeting your goals so can improve for the coming weeks. Don't get bogged down in minor setbacks or obstacles; instead, reward yourself for each small step of success along the way.

3 **Exercise Goals Wrap-Up:** Did you meet your exercise goals for the week? Why or why not? If you were happy with your physical activity for the week, give yourself a pat on the back. If you didn't meet your goals, assess how you can make positive changes the next week.

4 **Goals for Next Week:** This section helps motivate you for the week that is approaching. If you met your goal from the previous week, create a brand-new goal for the upcoming week. If you weren't successful in meeting your last goal, make it a priority to accomplish it in the upcoming week. Setting goals ahead of time means planning ahead for healthy meals and exercise.

MONTHLY PROGRESS PAGES

At the end of each month, record the date, your start and end weights, your body fat percentage, and your current measurements. If you have been successfully cutting calories, eating smart, exercising, drinking water and meeting your other goals you will be very pleased to see these numbers changing as you lose body fat and gain muscle. If your weight didn't drop as much as you would like, remember that if you are building muscle mass through an exercise plan, that may be a factor in your weight. While muscle weighs more than fat it also helps burn fat and calories more rapidly. Consider this, an additional two pounds of muscle burns up to 100 extra calories per day!

❶ Photo of the Month: Tape a photo of you here to visually track your weight-loss progress. You will love seeing how much thinner and more fit you look at the end of each month as you continue to track your daily intake and fitness.

❷ Highlight of the Month: The highlight of your month could be the amount of weight you lost or it could be meeting a goal, such as running a mile in a certain amount of time. Keeping track of your monthly milestones will keep you motivated and excited about your diet plan.

❸ Nutritional Intake Wrap-Up: At the end of each month, evaluate whether or not you were successful in meeting your monthly goals. For example, if one goal was to eat less fast-food and make dinner at home more in order to decrease your fat and calorie intake, describe what worked for you and what didn't. This helps you stay accountable, as well as reward yourself for a job well done when you meet your goals.

❹ Exercise Goals Wrap-Up: Did you meet your fitness goals for the month? If your answer is yes, congratulate yourself and keep it up. If your answer is no, evaluate what roadblocks and obstacles are getting in your way and find solutions. For example, if you don't feel you have enough time to exercise, consider building 30 minutes into your lunch break at work to go for a hike.

❺ Goals for Next Month: Planning ahead and having attainable goals is one of the keys to losing weight. Give yourself concrete milestones you can reach, such as cutting out all sweets except for a small treat you give yourself on Sundays. This gives you something to look forward to for the coming month.

MONTHLY

DATE:

02/05

START WEIGHT:

197

END WEIGHT:

192

BODY FAT %:

22

MEASUREMENTS:

44.5 chest

14.5 biceps

43 waist

43 hips

24.5 thighs

NOTES:

PHOTO OF THE MONTH

Photo comments.

Only a few more months until my vacation!

1

tape your photo here

PROGRESS

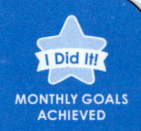

HIGHLIGHT OF THE MONTH

Your single-greatest moment of the month!

Going out with coworkers to happy hour and passing
on the nachos and hot wings!

2

NUTRITIONAL INTAKE WRAP-UP

Did you meet your intake goals for the month? Why or why not?

I did well except for drinking soda with lunch. That
is an easy place to cut a lot of calories and sugar.
I should be switching to water next month.

3

EXERCISE WRAP-UP

Did you meet your exercise goals for the month? Why or why not?

I got my mile time down. I can feel my endurance
building with each workout. I should drink more water
for more stamina.

4

GOALS FOR NEXT MONTH

Things to work on for next month.

My goal for next month is to wake up early and work
out on days I know I am busy after work.

I also want to cut back on drinking soda during
lunch. Switching to water will save hundreds of
calories.

5

NOTES

JOURNAL
PAGES

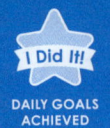
DATE:

3/2

WEIGHT:

223

WATER INTAKE:

# of 8oz. glasses

☑ ☐ ☐ ☐
☐ ☐ ☐ ☐

ENERGY LEVEL:

☐ low
☑ medium
☐ high

DAILY # OF SERVINGS:

fruits

veggies

grains

meats & beans

milk & dairy

oils & sweets

VITAMINS & SUPPLEMENTS:

DAILY NUTRITIONAL INTAKE

Food/Beverages	Qty.	Calories	Fat	Carbs.	Protein	Fiber
~~green smoothie~~						
lean shake		170	6	6	25	3

DAILY TOTALS:

DAILY EXERCISE

Activity	Hrs./Mins.	Cal. Burned
Treadmill	20	126

DAILY TOTALS:

TIP OF THE DAY!

Try not to eat while watching television, driving, reading or any other activity. It can make you lose track of how much you are eating.

DAILY NOTES, ACHIEVEMENTS

Obstacles, solutions, and thoughts on your progress.

TUESDAY

DAILY GOALS ACHIEVED

DAILY NUTRITIONAL INTAKE

Food/Beverages	Qty.	Calories	Fat	Carbs.	Protein	Fiber
_____	___					
_____	___					
_____	___					
_____	___					
_____	___					
_____	___					
_____	___					
_____	___					
_____	___					
_____	___					
_____	___					
_____	___					
_____	___					
_____	___					
_____	___					
_____	___					
DAILY TOTALS:						

DATE:

WEIGHT:

WATER INTAKE:
# of 8oz. glasses
☐ ☐ ☐ ☐
☐ ☐ ☐ ☐

ENERGY LEVEL:
☐ low
☐ medium
☐ high

DAILY # OF SERVINGS:
- fruits
- veggies
- grains
- meats & beans
- milk & dairy
- oils & sweets

VITAMINS & SUPPLEMENTS:

DAILY EXERCISE

Activity	Hrs./Mins.	Cal. Burned
_____	___	
_____	___	
_____	___	
_____	___	
DAILY TOTALS:		

TIP OF THE DAY!

Celebrate your success every day. Be proud of what you have accomplished and continue to envision the future you.

DAILY NOTES, ACHIEVEMENTS

Obstacles, solutions, and thoughts on your progress.

_____

_____

_____

I Did It!

DAILY GOALS
ACHIEVED

DATE:

WEIGHT:

WATER INTAKE:
# of 8oz. glasses

☐ ☐ ☐ ☐
☐ ☐ ☐ ☐

ENERGY LEVEL:
☐ low
☐ medium
☐ high

DAILY # OF SERVINGS:

fruits

veggies

grains

meats & beans

milk & dairy

oils & sweets

VITAMINS & SUPPLEMENTS:

DAILY NUTRITIONAL INTAKE

Food/Beverages	Qty.	Calories	Fat	Carbs.	Protein	Fiber
DAILY TOTALS:						

DAILY EXERCISE

Activity	Hrs./Mins.	Cal. Burned
DAILY TOTALS:		

TIP OF THE DAY!

Adding new food and variety to your plan will help keep your diet interesting and keep you motivated.

DAILY NOTES, ACHIEVEMENTS

Obstacles, solutions, and thoughts on your progress.

THURSDAY

I Did It!
DAILY GOALS ACHIEVED

DAILY NUTRITIONAL INTAKE

Food/Beverages	Qty.	Calories	Fat	Carbs.	Protein	Fiber
DAILY TOTALS:						

DAILY EXERCISE

Activity	Hrs./Mins.	Cal. Burned
DAILY TOTALS:		

TIP OF THE DAY!

Balance out a high-calorie breakfast by eating a moderate lunch and dinner.

DAILY NOTES, ACHIEVEMENTS

Obstacles, solutions, and thoughts on your progress.

DATE:

WEIGHT:

WATER INTAKE:
# of 8oz. glasses
☐ ☐ ☐ ☐
☐ ☐ ☐ ☐

ENERGY LEVEL:
☐ low
☐ medium
☐ high

DAILY # OF SERVINGS:
fruits
veggies
grains
meats & beans
milk & dairy
oils & sweets

VITAMINS & SUPPLEMENTS:

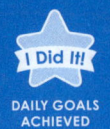

I Did It!

DAILY GOALS
ACHIEVED

WEEK
1

FRIDAY

DATE:

WEIGHT:

WATER INTAKE:
# of 8oz. glasses

☐ ☐ ☐ ☐
☐ ☐ ☐ ☐

ENERGY LEVEL:

☐ low
☐ medium
☐ high

DAILY # OF SERVINGS:

fruits

veggies

grains

meats & beans

milk & dairy

oils & sweets

VITAMINS & SUPPLEMENTS:

DAILY NUTRITIONAL INTAKE

Food/Beverages	Qty.	Calories	Fat	Carbs.	Protein	Fiber
DAILY TOTALS:						

DAILY EXERCISE

Activity	Hrs./Mins.	Cal. Burned
DAILY TOTALS:		

TIP OF THE DAY!

Disassociate diets with restriction and deprivation. Look at diets as eating the right foods in the right amounts.

DAILY NOTES, ACHIEVEMENTS

Obstacles, solutions, and thoughts on your progress.

SATURDAY

I Did It!

**DAILY GOALS
ACHIEVED**

DAILY NUTRITIONAL INTAKE

Food/Beverages	Qty.	Calories	Fat	Carbs.	Protein	Fiber
DAILY TOTALS:						

DATE:

WEIGHT:

WATER INTAKE:
# of 8oz. glasses

☐ ☑ ☐ ☐
☐ ☐ ☐ ☐

ENERGY LEVEL:
☐ low
☐ medium
☐ high

DAILY # OF SERVINGS:

fruits

veggies

grains

meats & beans

milk & dairy

oils & sweets

VITAMINS & SUPPLEMENTS:

DAILY EXERCISE

Activity	Hrs./Mins.	Cal. Burned
DAILY TOTALS:		

TIP OF THE DAY!

Don't be too hard on yourself if you stumble along the way. Just remind yourself that tomorrow is another day, and you can get back on track.

DAILY NOTES, ACHIEVEMENTS

Obstacles, solutions, and thoughts on your progress.

I Did It!
DAILY GOALS ACHIEVED

WEEK 1

SUNDAY

DATE:

WEIGHT:

WATER INTAKE:
# of 8oz. glasses

☐ ☐ ☐ ☐
☐ ☐ ☐ ☐

ENERGY LEVEL:

☐ low
☐ medium
☐ high

DAILY # OF SERVINGS:

fruits

veggies

grains

meats & beans

milk & dairy

oils & sweets

VITAMINS & SUPPLEMENTS:

DAILY NUTRITIONAL INTAKE

Food/Beverages	Qty.	Calories	Fat	Carbs.	Protein	Fiber
DAILY TOTALS:						

DAILY EXERCISE

Activity	Hrs./Mins.	Cal. Burned
DAILY TOTALS:		

TIP OF THE DAY!

The gratification of gradual weight loss will be much more satisfying than the instant gratification of food.

DAILY NOTES, ACHIEVEMENTS

Obstacles, solutions, and thoughts on your progress.

WEEKLY PROGRESS

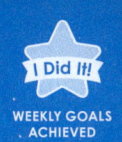

I Did It!

WEEKLY GOALS ACHIEVED

HIGHLIGHT OF THE WEEK

Your single-greatest moment of the week!

_____
_____
_____
_____

NUTRITIONAL INTAKE WRAP-UP

Did you meet your intake goals for the week? Why or why not?

_____
_____
_____
_____
_____
_____

EXERCISE WRAP-UP

Did you meet your exercise goals for the week? Why or why not?

_____
_____
_____
_____

GOALS FOR NEXT WEEK

Things to work on for next week.

_____
_____
_____
_____
_____
_____

START WEIGHT:

END WEIGHT:

DAYS I TRACKED MY DIET:
- ☐ Mon.
- ☐ Tues.
- ☐ Wed.
- ☐ Thurs.
- ☐ Fri.
- ☐ Sat.
- ☐ Sun.

DAYS I EXERCISED:
- ☐ Mon.
- ☐ Tues.
- ☐ Wed.
- ☐ Thurs.
- ☐ Fri.
- ☐ Sat.
- ☐ Sun.

WEEKLY CALORIES BURNED:

WEEKLY ENERGY LEVEL:
- ☐ low
- ☐ medium
- ☐ high

I Did It!
DAILY GOALS
ACHIEVED

DATE:

WEIGHT:

WATER INTAKE:
# of 8oz. glasses

☐ ☐ ☐ ☐
☐ ☐ ☐ ☐

ENERGY LEVEL:
☐ low
☐ medium
☐ high

DAILY # OF SERVINGS:

fruits

veggies

grains

meats & beans

milk & dairy

oils & sweets

VITAMINS & SUPPLEMENTS:

DAILY NUTRITIONAL INTAKE

Food/Beverages	Qty.	Calories	Fat	Carbs.	Protein	Fiber
DAILY TOTALS:						

DAILY EXERCISE

Activity	Hrs./Mins.	Cal. Burned
DAILY TOTALS:		

TIP OF THE DAY!

Set temporary or short-term goals for yourself. Breaking the journey down into smaller sections can make it easier to stay on track.

DAILY NOTES, ACHIEVEMENTS

Obstacles, solutions, and thoughts on your progress.

TUESDAY

I Did It!

DAILY GOALS ACHIEVED

DAILY NUTRITIONAL INTAKE

Food/Beverages	Qty.	Calories	Fat	Carbs.	Protein	Fiber
DAILY TOTALS:						

DAILY EXERCISE

Activity	Hrs./Mins.	Cal. Burned
DAILY TOTALS:		

TIP OF THE DAY!

Find a friend to share in your weight-loss journey— it can help you remain on track and stay motivated.

DAILY NOTES, ACHIEVEMENTS

Obstacles, solutions, and thoughts on your progress.

_____

_____

_____

DATE:

WEIGHT:

WATER INTAKE:
# of 8oz. glasses
☐ ☐ ☐ ☐
☐ ☐ ☐ ☐

ENERGY LEVEL:
☐ low
☐ medium
☐ high

DAILY # OF SERVINGS:
fruits
veggies
grains
meats & beans
milk & dairy
oils & sweets

VITAMINS & SUPPLEMENTS:

_____

_____

_____

_____

_____

_____

_____

I Did It!
DAILY GOALS
ACHIEVED

DATE:

WEIGHT:

WATER INTAKE:
# of 8oz. glasses

☐ ☐ ☐ ☐
☐ ☐ ☐ ☐

ENERGY LEVEL:

☐ low
☐ medium
☐ high

DAILY # OF SERVINGS:

fruits

veggies

grains

meats & beans

milk & dairy

oils & sweets

VITAMINS & SUPPLEMENTS:

DAILY NUTRITIONAL INTAKE

Food/Beverages	Qty.	Calories	Fat	Carbs.	Protein	Fiber
DAILY TOTALS:						

DAILY EXERCISE

Activity	Hrs./Mins.	Cal. Burned
DAILY TOTALS:		

TIP OF THE DAY!

Stick to your dietary commitment for at least 30 days. After the first 30 days, you will have practiced the behavior long enough to consider it a habit.

DAILY NOTES, ACHIEVEMENTS

Obstacles, solutions, and thoughts on your progress.

THURSDAY

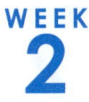

DAILY GOALS
ACHIEVED

DAILY NUTRITIONAL INTAKE

Food/Beverages	Qty.	Calories	Fat	Carbs.	Protein	Fiber
DAILY TOTALS:						

DAILY EXERCISE

Activity	Hrs./Mins.	Cal. Burned
DAILY TOTALS:		

TIP OF THE DAY!

Moderation is the key to a healthy lifestyle and to losing weight.

DAILY NOTES, ACHIEVEMENTS

Obstacles, solutions, and thoughts on your progress.

DATE:

WEIGHT:

WATER INTAKE:
# of 8oz. glasses

ENERGY LEVEL:
- [ ] low
- [ ] medium
- [ ] high

DAILY # OF SERVINGS:

fruits

veggies

grains

meats & beans

milk & dairy

oils & sweets

VITAMINS & SUPPLEMENTS:

I Did It!

DAILY GOALS
ACHIEVED

FRIDAY

DATE:

WEIGHT:

WATER INTAKE:
# of 8oz. glasses

☐ ☐ ☐ ☐
☐ ☐ ☐ ☐

ENERGY LEVEL:
☐ low
☐ medium
☐ high

DAILY # OF SERVINGS:

fruits

veggies

grains

meats & beans

milk & dairy

oils & sweets

VITAMINS & SUPPLEMENTS:

DAILY NUTRITIONAL INTAKE

Food/Beverages	Qty.	Calories	Fat	Carbs.	Protein	Fiber
DAILY TOTALS:						

DAILY EXERCISE

Activity	Hrs./Mins.	Cal. Burned
DAILY TOTALS:		

TIP OF THE DAY!

Order a sandwich with whole grain bread instead of white.

DAILY NOTES, ACHIEVEMENTS

Obstacles, solutions, and thoughts on your progress.

SATURDAY

I Did It!

DAILY GOALS ACHIEVED

DAILY NUTRITIONAL INTAKE

Food/Beverages	Qty.	Calories	Fat	Carbs.	Protein	Fiber
DAILY TOTALS:						

DAILY EXERCISE

Activity	Hrs./Mins.	Cal. Burned
DAILY TOTALS:		

TIP OF THE DAY!

Incorporate foods from each of the 6 main food groups into your diet plan.

DAILY NOTES, ACHIEVEMENTS

Obstacles, solutions, and thoughts on your progress.

_____
_____
_____

DATE:

WEIGHT:

WATER INTAKE:
# of 8oz. glasses
☐ ☐ ☐ ☐
☐ ☐ ☐ ☐

ENERGY LEVEL:
☐ low
☐ medium
☐ high

DAILY # OF SERVINGS:

fruits

veggies

grains

meats & beans

milk & dairy

oils & sweets

VITAMINS & SUPPLEMENTS:

_____
_____
_____
_____
_____
_____
_____
_____

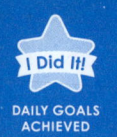

I Did It!
DAILY GOALS
ACHIEVED

WEEK 2

SUNDAY

DATE:

WEIGHT:

WATER INTAKE:
# of 8oz. glasses

☐ ☐ ☐ ☐
☐ ☐ ☐ ☐

ENERGY LEVEL:
☐ low
☐ medium
☐ high

DAILY # OF SERVINGS:

fruits

veggies

grains

meats & beans

milk & dairy

oils & sweets

VITAMINS & SUPPLEMENTS:

DAILY NUTRITIONAL INTAKE

Food/Beverages	Qty.	Calories	Fat	Carbs.	Protein	Fiber
DAILY TOTALS:						

DAILY EXERCISE

Activity	Hrs./Mins.	Cal. Burned
DAILY TOTALS:		

TIP OF THE DAY!

Drink plenty of water each day. Often we think we are hungry when our body is sending us signals that we are actually thirsty or dehydrated.

DAILY NOTES, ACHIEVEMENTS

Obstacles, solutions, and thoughts on your progress.

WEEKLY PROGRESS

WEEK 2

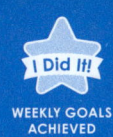

I Did It!

WEEKLY GOALS ACHIEVED

HIGHLIGHT OF THE WEEK

Your single-greatest moment of the week!

_____
_____
_____
_____
_____

NUTRITIONAL INTAKE WRAP-UP

Did you meet your intake goals for the week? Why or why not?

_____
_____
_____
_____
_____
_____

EXERCISE WRAP-UP

Did you meet your exercise goals for the week? Why or why not?

_____
_____
_____
_____
_____

GOALS FOR NEXT WEEK

Things to work on for next week.

_____
_____
_____
_____
_____
_____
_____
_____

START WEIGHT:

END WEIGHT:

DAYS I TRACKED MY DIET:

☐ Mon.
☐ Tues.
☐ Wed.
☐ Thurs.
☐ Fri.
☐ Sat.
☐ Sun.

DAYS I EXERCISED:

☐ Mon.
☐ Tues.
☐ Wed.
☐ Thurs.
☐ Fri.
☐ Sat.
☐ Sun.

WEEKLY CALORIES BURNED:

WEEKLY ENERGY LEVEL:

☐ low
☐ medium
☐ high

I Did It!
DAILY GOALS
ACHIEVED

DATE:

WEIGHT:

WATER INTAKE:
# of 8oz. glasses

☐ ☐ ☐ ☐
☐ ☐ ☐ ☐

ENERGY LEVEL:
☐ low
☐ medium
☐ high

DAILY # OF SERVINGS:

fruits

veggies

grains

meats & beans

milk & dairy

oils & sweets

VITAMINS & SUPPLEMENTS:

DAILY NUTRITIONAL INTAKE

Food/Beverages	Qty.	Calories	Fat	Carbs.	Protein	Fiber

DAILY TOTALS:

DAILY EXERCISE

Activity	Hrs./Mins.	Cal. Burned

DAILY TOTALS:

TIP OF THE DAY!

Get adequate vitamins and minerals by eating a wide variety of fruits and vegetables.

DAILY NOTES, ACHIEVEMENTS

Obstacles, solutions, and thoughts on your progress.

TUESDAY

WEEK **3**

I Did It!

DAILY GOALS ACHIEVED

DAILY NUTRITIONAL INTAKE

Food/Beverages	Qty.	Calories	Fat	Carbs.	Protein	Fiber
_____	_____					
_____	_____					
_____	_____					
_____	_____					
_____	_____					
_____	_____					
_____	_____					
_____	_____					
_____	_____					
_____	_____					
_____	_____					
_____	_____					
_____	_____					
_____	_____					
_____	_____					
_____	_____					
_____	_____					
DAILY TOTALS:						

DAILY EXERCISE

Activity	Hrs./Mins.	Cal. Burned
_____	_____	
_____	_____	
_____	_____	
_____	_____	
DAILY TOTALS:		

TIP OF THE DAY!

Complex carbohydrates are crucial for losing weight as well as for maintaining energy.

DAILY NOTES, ACHIEVEMENTS

Obstacles, solutions, and thoughts on your progress.

_____

_____

_____

DATE:

WEIGHT:

WATER INTAKE:
# of 8oz. glasses

☐ ☐ ☐ ☐
☐ ☐ ☐ ☐

ENERGY LEVEL:

☐ low
☐ medium
☐ high

DAILY # OF SERVINGS:

fruits

veggies

grains

meats & beans

milk & dairy

oils & sweets

VITAMINS & SUPPLEMENTS:

_____

_____

_____

_____

_____

I Did It!

DAILY GOALS
ACHIEVED

WEEK 3 WEDNESDAY

DATE:

WEIGHT:

WATER INTAKE:
# of 8oz. glasses

☐ ☐ ☐ ☐
☐ ☐ ☐ ☐

ENERGY LEVEL:
☐ low
☐ medium
☐ high

DAILY # OF SERVINGS:

fruits

veggies

grains

meats & beans

milk & dairy

oils & sweets

VITAMINS & SUPPLEMENTS:

_____
_____
_____
_____
_____

DAILY NUTRITIONAL INTAKE

Food/Beverages	Qty.	Calories	Fat	Carbs.	Protein	Fiber

DAILY TOTALS:

DAILY EXERCISE

Activity	Hrs./Mins.	Cal. Burned

DAILY TOTALS:

TIP OF THE DAY!

Diets that rely on "tricks" are difficult to maintain and can damage your body. Learn how to distinguish a fad diet from a sensible one.

DAILY NOTES, ACHIEVEMENTS

Obstacles, solutions, and thoughts on your progress.

_____
_____
_____

THURSDAY

 I Did It!

DAILY GOALS ACHIEVED

DAILY NUTRITIONAL INTAKE

Food/Beverages	Qty.	Calories	Fat	Carbs.	Protein	Fiber
DAILY TOTALS:						

DAILY EXERCISE

Activity	Hrs./Mins.	Cal. Burned
DAILY TOTALS:		

TIP OF THE DAY!

Give yourself a planned break from your diet every once in a while. Figure out what you can enjoy without undermining your weight loss.

DAILY NOTES, ACHIEVEMENTS

Obstacles, solutions, and thoughts on your progress.

DATE:

WEIGHT:

WATER INTAKE:
# of 8oz. glasses

☐ ☐ ☐ ☐
☐ ☐ ☐ ☐

ENERGY LEVEL:

☐ low
☐ medium
☐ high

DAILY # OF SERVINGS:

fruits

veggies

grains

meats & beans

milk & dairy

oils & sweets

VITAMINS & SUPPLEMENTS:

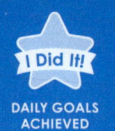

I Did It!
DAILY GOALS ACHIEVED

WEEK
3

FRIDAY

DATE:

WEIGHT:

WATER INTAKE:
# of 8oz. glasses

☐ ☐ ☐ ☐
☐ ☐ ☐ ☐

ENERGY LEVEL:

☐ low
☐ medium
☐ high

DAILY # OF SERVINGS:

fruits

veggies

grains

meats & beans

milk & dairy

oils & sweets

VITAMINS & SUPPLEMENTS:

_____
_____
_____
_____
_____

DAILY NUTRITIONAL INTAKE

Food/Beverages	Qty.	Calories	Fat	Carbs.	Protein	Fiber
DAILY TOTALS:						

DAILY EXERCISE

Activity	Hrs./Mins.	Cal. Burned
DAILY TOTALS:		

TIP OF THE DAY!

Try to eat several hours before going to bed so your body has a chance to burn off extra calories.

DAILY NOTES, ACHIEVEMENTS

Obstacles, solutions, and thoughts on your progress.

SATURDAY

DAILY GOALS
ACHIEVED

DAILY NUTRITIONAL INTAKE

Food/Beverages	Qty.	Calories	Fat	Carbs.	Protein	Fiber
_____	____					
_____	____					
_____	____					
_____	____					
_____	____					
_____	____					
_____	____					
_____	____					
_____	____					
_____	____					
_____	____					
_____	____					
_____	____					
_____	____					
_____	____					
_____	____					
DAILY TOTALS:						

DAILY EXERCISE

Activity	Hrs./Mins.	Cal. Burned
_____	_____	
_____	_____	
_____	_____	
_____	_____	
_____	_____	
DAILY TOTALS:		

TIP OF THE DAY!

Eat fewer carbohydrates, such as white bread, chips and cookies, at nighttime.

DAILY NOTES, ACHIEVEMENTS

Obstacles, solutions, and thoughts on your progress.

_____

_____

_____

DATE:

WEIGHT:

WATER INTAKE:
# of 8oz. glasses
☐ ☐ ☐ ☐
☐ ☐ ☐ ☐

ENERGY LEVEL:
☐ low
☐ medium
☐ high

DAILY # OF SERVINGS:

fruits

veggies

grains

meats & beans

milk & dairy

oils & sweets

VITAMINS & SUPPLEMENTS:

_____

_____

_____

_____

_____

_____

I Did It!
DAILY GOALS
ACHIEVED

WEEK
3

SUNDAY

DATE:

WEIGHT:

WATER INTAKE:
# of 8oz. glasses

☐ ☐ ☐ ☐
☐ ☐ ☐ ☐

ENERGY LEVEL:
☐ low
☐ medium
☐ high

DAILY # OF SERVINGS:

fruits

veggies

grains

meats & beans

milk & dairy

oils & sweets

VITAMINS & SUPPLEMENTS:

DAILY NUTRITIONAL INTAKE

Food/Beverages	Qty.	Calories	Fat	Carbs.	Protein	Fiber
DAILY TOTALS:						

DAILY EXERCISE

Activity	Hrs./Mins.	Cal. Burned
DAILY TOTALS:		

TIP OF THE DAY!

Make your weight-loss goals reasonable and reachable; that way you will be more likely to reach them and achieve your resolutions.

DAILY NOTES, ACHIEVEMENTS

Obstacles, solutions, and thoughts on your progress.

WEEKLY PROGRESS

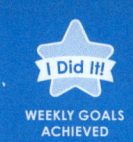

I Did It!

WEEKLY GOALS ACHIEVED

HIGHLIGHT OF THE WEEK

Your single-greatest moment of the week!

_____

_____

_____

_____

START WEIGHT:

END WEIGHT:

NUTRITIONAL INTAKE WRAP-UP

Did you meet your intake goals for the week? Why or why not?

_____

_____

_____

_____

_____

_____

DAYS I TRACKED MY DIET:

☐ Mon.

☐ Tues.

☐ Wed.

☐ Thurs.

☐ Fri.

☐ Sat.

☐ Sun.

EXERCISE WRAP-UP

Did you meet your exercise goals for the week? Why or why not?

_____

_____

_____

_____

_____

DAYS I EXERCISED:

☐ Mon.

☐ Tues.

☐ Wed.

☐ Thurs.

☐ Fri.

☐ Sat.

☐ Sun.

GOALS FOR NEXT WEEK

Things to work on for next week.

_____

_____

_____

_____

_____

_____

_____

WEEKLY CALORIES BURNED:

WEEKLY ENERGY LEVEL:

☐ low

☐ medium

☐ high

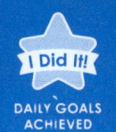

I Did It!
DAILY GOALS
ACHIEVED

DATE:

WEIGHT:

WATER INTAKE:
# of 8oz. glasses

☐ ☐ ☐ ☐
☐ ☐ ☐ ☐

ENERGY LEVEL:
☐ low
☐ medium
☐ high

DAILY # OF SERVINGS:

fruits

veggies

grains

meats & beans

milk & dairy

oils & sweets

VITAMINS & SUPPLEMENTS:

DAILY NUTRITIONAL INTAKE

Food/Beverages	Qty.	Calories	Fat	Carbs.	Protein	Fiber
DAILY TOTALS:						

DAILY EXERCISE

Activity	Hrs./Mins.	Cal. Burned
DAILY TOTALS:		

TIP OF THE DAY!

Take into account your age and health status. Understand what your body needs before coming up with an appropriate weight-loss program.

DAILY NOTES, ACHIEVEMENTS

Obstacles, solutions, and thoughts on your progress.

TUESDAY

I Did It!

DAILY GOALS ACHIEVED

DAILY NUTRITIONAL INTAKE

Food/Beverages	Qty.	Calories	Fat	Carbs.	Protein	Fiber
_____	___					
_____	___					
_____	___					
_____	___					
_____	___					
_____	___					
_____	___					
_____	___					
_____	___					
_____	___					
_____	___					
_____	___					
_____	___					
_____	___					
_____	___					
_____	___					
_____	___					
DAILY TOTALS:						

DAILY EXERCISE

Activity	Hrs./Mins.	Cal. Burned
_____	_____	
_____	_____	
_____	_____	
_____	_____	
_____	_____	
DAILY TOTALS:		

TIP OF THE DAY!

Knowing the effects of every diet, and whether or not there are any downsides, will help you make the correct decision.

DAILY NOTES, ACHIEVEMENTS

Obstacles, solutions, and thoughts on your progress.

_____
_____
_____

DATE:

WEIGHT:

WATER INTAKE:
# of 8oz. glasses
☐ ☐ ☐ ☐
☐ ☐ ☐ ☐

ENERGY LEVEL:
☐ low
☐ medium
☐ high

DAILY # OF SERVINGS:

fruits

veggies

grains

meats & beans

milk & dairy

oils & sweets

VITAMINS & SUPPLEMENTS:

_____
_____
_____
_____
_____
_____

I Did It!

DAILY GOALS ACHIEVED

WEEK
4

WEDNESDAY

DATE:

WEIGHT:

WATER INTAKE:
# of 8oz. glasses

☐ ☐ ☐ ☐
☐ ☐ ☐ ☐

ENERGY LEVEL:

☐ low
☐ medium
☐ high

DAILY # OF SERVINGS:

fruits

veggies

grains

meats & beans

milk & dairy

oils & sweets

VITAMINS & SUPPLEMENTS:

DAILY NUTRITIONAL INTAKE

Food/Beverages	Qty.	Calories	Fat	Carbs.	Protein	Fiber
DAILY TOTALS:						

DAILY EXERCISE

Activity	Hrs./Mins.	Cal. Burned
DAILY TOTALS:		

TIP OF THE DAY!

Get lots of sleep. Lack of sleep can lead to an increase in appetite, including cravings for fatty and sugary foods.

DAILY NOTES, ACHIEVEMENTS

Obstacles, solutions, and thoughts on your progress.

THURSDAY

I Did It!

**DAILY GOALS
ACHIEVED**

DAILY NUTRITIONAL INTAKE

Food/Beverages	Qty.	Calories	Fat	Carbs.	Protein	Fiber
DAILY TOTALS:						

DAILY EXERCISE

Activity	Hrs./Mins.	Cal. Burned
DAILY TOTALS:		

TIP OF THE DAY!

Whole grains are very beneficial to your body. They can help reduce the risk of high cholesterol or blood pressure, diabetes, and certain heart diseases.

DAILY NOTES, ACHIEVEMENTS

Obstacles, solutions, and thoughts on your progress.

DATE:

WEIGHT:

WATER INTAKE:
# of 8oz. glasses

☐ ☐ ☐ ☐
☐ ☐ ☐ ☐

ENERGY LEVEL:

☐ low

☐ medium

☐ high

DAILY # OF SERVINGS:

fruits

veggies

grains

meats & beans

milk & dairy

oils & sweets

VITAMINS & SUPPLEMENTS:

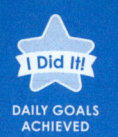
DATE:

WEIGHT:

WATER INTAKE:

# of 8oz. glasses

☐ ☐ ☐ ☐
☐ ☐ ☐ ☐

ENERGY LEVEL:

☐ low
☐ medium
☐ high

DAILY # OF SERVINGS:

fruits

veggies

grains

meats & beans

milk & dairy

oils & sweets

VITAMINS & SUPPLEMENTS:

DAILY NUTRITIONAL INTAKE

Food/Beverages	Qty.	Calories	Fat	Carbs.	Protein	Fiber
DAILY TOTALS:						

DAILY EXERCISE

Activity	Hrs./Mins.	Cal. Burned
DAILY TOTALS:		

TIP OF THE DAY!

Avoid foods with trans fats, such as candy, chips, packaged snacks, pastries, donuts, cookies and fried foods.

DAILY NOTES, ACHIEVEMENTS

Obstacles, solutions, and thoughts on your progress.

SATURDAY

DAILY GOALS
ACHIEVED

DAILY NUTRITIONAL INTAKE

Food/Beverages	Qty.	Calories	Fat	Carbs.	Protein	Fiber
_____	___					
_____	___					
_____	___					
_____	___					
_____	___					
_____	___					
_____	___					
_____	___					
_____	___					
_____	___					
_____	___					
_____	___					
_____	___					
_____	___					
_____	___					
_____	___					
DAILY TOTALS:						

DAILY EXERCISE

Activity	Hrs./Mins.	Cal. Burned
_____	_____	
_____	_____	
_____	_____	
_____	_____	
_____	_____	
DAILY TOTALS:		

TIP OF THE DAY!

Achieving a healthy
lifestyle takes time
and practice, but you
can do it.

DAILY NOTES, ACHIEVEMENTS

Obstacles, solutions, and thoughts on your progress.

_____

_____

_____

DATE:

WEIGHT:

WATER INTAKE:
# of 8oz. glasses

☐ ☐ ☐ ☐
☐ ☐ ☐ ☐

ENERGY LEVEL:

☐ low

☐ medium

☐ high

DAILY # OF SERVINGS:

fruits

veggies

grains

meats &
beans

milk &
dairy

oils &
sweets

**VITAMINS &
SUPPLEMENTS:**

_____

_____

_____

_____

_____

_____

_____

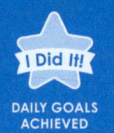

I Did It!
DAILY GOALS
ACHIEVED

DATE:

WEIGHT:

WATER INTAKE:
# of 8oz. glasses

☐ ☐ ☐ ☐
☐ ☐ ☐ ☐

ENERGY LEVEL:
☐ low
☐ medium
☐ high

DAILY # OF SERVINGS:

fruits

veggies

grains

meats & beans

milk & dairy

oils & sweets

VITAMINS & SUPPLEMENTS:

DAILY NUTRITIONAL INTAKE

Food/Beverages	Qty.	Calories	Fat	Carbs.	Protein	Fiber
DAILY TOTALS:						

DAILY EXERCISE

Activity	Hrs./Mins.	Cal. Burned
DAILY TOTALS:		

TIP OF THE DAY!

Keep physical fitness a priority through exercise routines that are realistic, maintainable, and fun.

DAILY NOTES, ACHIEVEMENTS

Obstacles, solutions, and thoughts on your progress.

WEEKLY PROGRESS

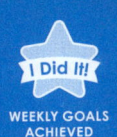

I Did It!

WEEKLY GOALS ACHIEVED

HIGHLIGHT OF THE WEEK

Your single-greatest moment of the week!

_____

_____

_____

_____

NUTRITIONAL INTAKE WRAP-UP

Did you meet your intake goals for the week? Why or why not?

_____

_____

_____

_____

_____

_____

_____

EXERCISE WRAP-UP

Did you meet your exercise goals for the week? Why or why not?

_____

_____

_____

_____

GOALS FOR NEXT WEEK

Things to work on for next week.

_____

_____

_____

_____

_____

_____

_____

_____

START WEIGHT:

END WEIGHT:

DAYS I TRACKED MY DIET:
- ☐ Mon.
- ☐ Tues.
- ☐ Wed.
- ☐ Thurs.
- ☐ Fri.
- ☐ Sat.
- ☐ Sun.

DAYS I EXERCISED:
- ☐ Mon.
- ☐ Tues.
- ☐ Wed.
- ☐ Thurs.
- ☐ Fri.
- ☐ Sat.
- ☐ Sun.

WEEKLY CALORIES BURNED:

WEEKLY ENERGY LEVEL:
- ☐ low
- ☐ medium
- ☐ high

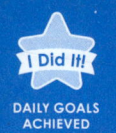

I Did It!
DAILY GOALS
ACHIEVED

WEEK
5

MONDAY

DATE:

WEIGHT:

WATER INTAKE:
# of 8oz. glasses

☐ ☐ ☐ ☐
☐ ☐ ☐ ☐

ENERGY LEVEL:
☐ low
☐ medium
☐ high

DAILY # OF SERVINGS:

fruits

veggies

grains

meats & beans

milk & dairy

oils & sweets

VITAMINS & SUPPLEMENTS:

DAILY NUTRITIONAL INTAKE

Food/Beverages	Qty.	Calories	Fat	Carbs.	Protein	Fiber
DAILY TOTALS:						

DAILY EXERCISE

Activity	Hrs./Mins.	Cal. Burned
DAILY TOTALS:		

TIP OF THE DAY!

Avoid high-fructose corn syrup, found in sweets and other processed foods like condiments, salad dressing, canned fruit, and soups.

DAILY NOTES, ACHIEVEMENTS

Obstacles, solutions, and thoughts on your progress.

TUESDAY

I Did It!

DAILY GOALS
ACHIEVED

DAILY NUTRITIONAL INTAKE

Food/Beverages	Qty.	Calories	Fat	Carbs.	Protein	Fiber
DAILY TOTALS:						

DAILY EXERCISE

Activity	Hrs./Mins.	Cal. Burned
DAILY TOTALS:		

TIP OF THE DAY!

If you cannot make it to the gym every day, try to incorporate other physical activities into your day, such as gardening, vacuuming, or shopping.

DAILY NOTES, ACHIEVEMENTS

Obstacles, solutions, and thoughts on your progress.

DATE:

WEIGHT:

WATER INTAKE:
# of 8oz. glasses
☐ ☐ ☐ ☐
☐ ☐ ☐ ☐

ENERGY LEVEL:
☐ low
☐ medium
☐ high

DAILY # OF SERVINGS:

fruits

veggies

grains

meats & beans

milk & dairy

oils & sweets

VITAMINS & SUPPLEMENTS:

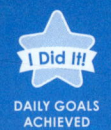

I Did It!

DAILY GOALS
ACHIEVED

WEEK
5

WEDNESDAY

DATE:

WEIGHT:

WATER INTAKE:
# of 8oz. glasses

☐ ☐ ☐ ☐
☐ ☐ ☐ ☐

ENERGY LEVEL:
☐ low
☐ medium
☐ high

DAILY # OF SERVINGS:

fruits

veggies

grains

meats & beans

milk & dairy

oils & sweets

VITAMINS & SUPPLEMENTS:

DAILY NUTRITIONAL INTAKE

Food/Beverages	Qty.	Calories	Fat	Carbs.	Protein	Fiber
DAILY TOTALS:						

DAILY EXERCISE

Activity	Hrs./Mins.	Cal. Burned
DAILY TOTALS:		

TIP OF THE DAY!

Occasionally get up from your desk and stretch. Take every opportunity to add movement to your day.

DAILY NOTES, ACHIEVEMENTS

Obstacles, solutions, and thoughts on your progress.

THURSDAY

I Did It!

DAILY GOALS
ACHIEVED

DAILY NUTRITIONAL INTAKE

Food/Beverages	Qty.	Calories	Fat	Carbs.	Protein	Fiber
_____	_____					
_____	_____					
_____	_____					
_____	_____					
_____	_____					
_____	_____					
_____	_____					
_____	_____					
_____	_____					
_____	_____					
_____	_____					
_____	_____					
_____	_____					
_____	_____					
_____	_____					
_____	_____					
_____	_____					
DAILY TOTALS:						

DATE:

WEIGHT:

WATER INTAKE:
# of 8oz. glasses
☐ ☐ ☐ ☐
☐ ☐ ☐ ☐

ENERGY LEVEL:
☐ low
☐ medium
☐ high

DAILY # OF SERVINGS:

fruits

veggies

grains

meats & beans

milk & dairy

oils & sweets

VITAMINS & SUPPLEMENTS:

_____

_____

_____

_____

_____

_____

_____

DAILY EXERCISE

Activity	Hrs./Mins.	Cal. Burned
_____	_____	
_____	_____	
_____	_____	
_____	_____	
_____	_____	
DAILY TOTALS:		

TIP OF THE DAY!

When dining out, be aware of hidden calories, sodium, and fats that could be included in sauces or the way the meals are prepared in the kitchen.

DAILY NOTES, ACHIEVEMENTS

Obstacles, solutions, and thoughts on your progress.

_____

_____

_____

I Did It!

DAILY GOALS ACHIEVED

WEEK
5

FRIDAY

DATE:

WEIGHT:

WATER INTAKE:
# of 8oz. glasses

☐ ☐ ☐ ☐
☐ ☐ ☐ ☐

ENERGY LEVEL:
☐ low
☐ medium
☐ high

DAILY # OF SERVINGS:

fruits

veggies

grains

meats & beans

milk & dairy

oils & sweets

VITAMINS & SUPPLEMENTS:

DAILY NUTRITIONAL INTAKE

Food/Beverages	Qty.	Calories	Fat	Carbs.	Protein	Fiber
DAILY TOTALS:						

DAILY EXERCISE

Activity	Hrs./Mins.	Cal. Burned
DAILY TOTALS:		

TIP OF THE DAY!

Don't be afraid to ask your server how the meal is prepared, or to request that the food be prepared in a way that is in keeping with your diet program.

DAILY NOTES, ACHIEVEMENTS

Obstacles, solutions, and thoughts on your progress.

SATURDAY

DAILY NUTRITIONAL INTAKE

Food/Beverages	Qty.	Calories	Fat	Carbs.	Protein	Fiber
_____	____					
_____	____					
_____	____					
_____	____					
_____	____					
_____	____					
_____	____					
_____	____					
_____	____					
_____	____					
_____	____					
_____	____					
_____	____					
_____	____					
DAILY TOTALS:						

DATE:

WEIGHT:

WATER INTAKE:
# of 8oz. glasses
☐ ☐ ☐ ☐
☐ ☐ ☐ ☐

ENERGY LEVEL:
☐ low
☐ medium
☐ high

DAILY # OF SERVINGS:

fruits

veggies

grains

meats & beans

milk & dairy

oils & sweets

VITAMINS & SUPPLEMENTS:

_____
_____
_____
_____
_____
_____
_____

DAILY EXERCISE

Activity	Hrs./Mins.	Cal. Burned
_____	_____	
_____	_____	
_____	_____	
_____	_____	
_____	_____	
DAILY TOTALS:		

TIP OF THE DAY!

Try to eat only part of what is on your plate and eat the rest as leftovers the next day.

DAILY NOTES, ACHIEVEMENTS

Obstacles, solutions, and thoughts on your progress.

_____
_____
_____
_____

I Did It!

DAILY GOALS
ACHIEVED

DATE:

WEIGHT:

WATER INTAKE:
# of 8oz. glasses

☐ ☐ ☐ ☐
☐ ☐ ☐ ☐

ENERGY LEVEL:

☐ low
☐ medium
☐ high

DAILY # OF SERVINGS:

fruits

veggies

grains

meats & beans

milk & dairy

oils & sweets

VITAMINS & SUPPLEMENTS:

DAILY NUTRITIONAL INTAKE							
Food/Beverages	Qty.	Calories	Fat	Carbs.	Protein	Fiber
DAILY TOTALS:							

DAILY EXERCISE		
Activity	Hrs./Mins.	Cal. Burned
DAILY TOTALS:		

TIP OF THE DAY!

Read Nutritional Facts Labels to help you measure out correct serving sizes so you don't overeat.

DAILY NOTES, ACHIEVEMENTS

Obstacles, solutions, and thoughts on your progress.

WEEKLY PROGRESS

WEEK 5

 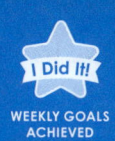

WEEKLY GOALS ACHIEVED

HIGHLIGHT OF THE WEEK

Your single-greatest moment of the week!

_____
_____
_____
_____
_____

START WEIGHT:

END WEIGHT:

NUTRITIONAL INTAKE WRAP-UP

Did you meet your intake goals for the week? Why or why not?

_____
_____
_____
_____
_____
_____
_____

DAYS I TRACKED MY DIET:

☐ Mon.
☐ Tues.
☐ Wed.
☐ Thurs.
☐ Fri.
☐ Sat.
☐ Sun.

EXERCISE WRAP-UP

Did you meet your exercise goals for the week? Why or why not?

_____
_____
_____
_____
_____

DAYS I EXERCISED:

☐ Mon.
☐ Tues.
☐ Wed.
☐ Thurs.
☐ Fri.
☐ Sat.
☐ Sun.

GOALS FOR NEXT WEEK

Things to work on for next week.

_____
_____
_____
_____
_____
_____
_____

WEEKLY CALORIES BURNED:

WEEKLY ENERGY LEVEL:

☐ low
☐ medium
☐ high

MONTHLY

DATE:

START WEIGHT:

END WEIGHT:

BODY FAT %:

MEASUREMENTS:

chest

biceps

waist

hips

thighs

NOTES:

PHOTO OF THE MONTH

Photo comments.

tape your photo here

PROGRESS

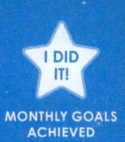

I DID IT!

MONTHLY GOALS ACHIEVED

HIGHLIGHT OF THE MONTH

Your single-greatest moment of the month!

_____

_____

_____

_____

NUTRITIONAL INTAKE WRAP-UP

Did you meet your intake goals for the month? Why or why not?

_____

_____

_____

_____

_____

_____

_____

EXERCISE WRAP-UP

Did you meet your exercise goals for the month? Why or why not?

_____

_____

_____

_____

GOALS FOR NEXT MONTH

Things to work on for next month.

_____

_____

_____

_____

_____

_____

_____

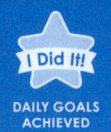

I Did It!
DAILY GOALS
ACHIEVED

WEEK
6

MONDAY

DATE:

WEIGHT:

WATER INTAKE:
# of 8oz. glasses

☐ ☐ ☐ ☐
☐ ☐ ☐ ☐

ENERGY LEVEL:
☐ low
☐ medium
☐ high

DAILY # OF SERVINGS:

fruits

veggies

grains

meats & beans

milk & dairy

oils & sweets

VITAMINS & SUPPLEMENTS:

DAILY NUTRITIONAL INTAKE

Food/Beverages	Qty.	Calories	Fat	Carbs.	Protein	Fiber
DAILY TOTALS:						

DAILY EXERCISE

Activity	Hrs./Mins.	Cal. Burned
DAILY TOTALS:		

TIP OF THE DAY!

If having a party, try to provide low-calorie, healthy snacks like vegetables and dip, baked potato chips, fruit slices, and water.

DAILY NOTES, ACHIEVEMENTS

Obstacles, solutions, and thoughts on your progress.

TUESDAY

I Did It!

DAILY GOALS ACHIEVED

DAILY NUTRITIONAL INTAKE

Food/Beverages	Qty.	Calories	Fat	Carbs.	Protein	Fiber
_____	_____					
_____	_____					
_____	_____					
_____	_____					
_____	_____					
_____	_____					
_____	_____					
_____	_____					
_____	_____					
_____	_____					
_____	_____					
_____	_____					
_____	_____					
_____	_____					
_____	_____					
_____	_____					
_____	_____					
DAILY TOTALS:						

DATE:

WEIGHT:

WATER INTAKE:
# of 8oz. glasses

☐ ☐ ☐ ☐
☐ ☐ ☐ ☐

ENERGY LEVEL:

☐ low
☐ medium
☐ high

DAILY # OF SERVINGS:

fruits

veggies

grains

meats & beans

milk & dairy

oils & sweets

VITAMINS & SUPPLEMENTS:

_____
_____
_____
_____
_____
_____

DAILY EXERCISE

Activity	Hrs./Mins.	Cal. Burned
_____	_____	
_____	_____	
_____	_____	
_____	_____	
DAILY TOTALS:		

TIP OF THE DAY!

Consult a registered dietician, a highly trained food and nutrition expert, who can help you with your nutrition questions.

DAILY NOTES, ACHIEVEMENTS

Obstacles, solutions, and thoughts on your progress.

_____

_____

_____

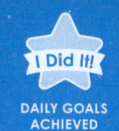

I Did It!

DAILY GOALS
ACHIEVED

WEEK 6

WEDNESDAY

DATE:

WEIGHT:

WATER INTAKE:
# of 8oz. glasses

☐ ☐ ☐ ☐
☐ ☐ ☐ ☐

ENERGY LEVEL:

☐ low
☐ medium
☐ high

DAILY # OF SERVINGS:

fruits

veggies

grains

meats & beans

milk & dairy

oils & sweets

VITAMINS & SUPPLEMENTS:

DAILY NUTRITIONAL INTAKE

Food/Beverages	Qty.	Calories	Fat	Carbs.	Protein	Fiber
DAILY TOTALS:						

DAILY EXERCISE

Activity	Hrs./Mins.	Cal. Burned
DAILY TOTALS:		

TIP OF THE DAY!

Get moving: An active person burns approximately 30 percent of their calories through daily non-exercise activity, versus 15 percent for sedentary people.

DAILY NOTES, ACHIEVEMENTS

Obstacles, solutions, and thoughts on your progress.

THURSDAY

I Did It!

DAILY GOALS ACHIEVED

DAILY NUTRITIONAL INTAKE

Food/Beverages	Qty.	Calories	Fat	Carbs.	Protein	Fiber
DAILY TOTALS:						

DAILY EXERCISE

Activity	Hrs./Mins.	Cal. Burned
DAILY TOTALS:		

TIP OF THE DAY!

Weight loss will help lower your risk of certain diseases, improve your overall health, and build your self-confidence.

DAILY NOTES, ACHIEVEMENTS

Obstacles, solutions, and thoughts on your progress.

DATE:

WEIGHT:

WATER INTAKE:
# of 8oz. glasses
☐ ☐ ☐ ☐
☐ ☐ ☐ ☐

ENERGY LEVEL:
☐ low
☐ medium
☐ high

DAILY # OF SERVINGS:

fruits

veggies

grains

meats & beans

milk & dairy

oils & sweets

VITAMINS & SUPPLEMENTS:

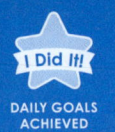

I Did It!
DAILY GOALS
ACHIEVED

WEEK
6

FRIDAY

DATE:

WEIGHT:

WATER INTAKE:
# of 8oz. glasses

☐ ☐ ☐ ☐
☐ ☐ ☐ ☐

ENERGY LEVEL:
☐ low
☐ medium
☐ high

DAILY # OF SERVINGS:

fruits

veggies

grains

meats & beans

milk & dairy

oils & sweets

VITAMINS & SUPPLEMENTS:

DAILY NUTRITIONAL INTAKE

Food/Beverages	Qty.	Calories	Fat	Carbs.	Protein	Fiber
DAILY TOTALS:						

DAILY EXERCISE

Activity	Hrs./Mins.	Cal. Burned
DAILY TOTALS:		

TIP OF THE DAY!

Stay hydrated: Water enables your body to work effectively at burning stored fat.

DAILY NOTES, ACHIEVEMENTS

Obstacles, solutions, and thoughts on your progress.

SATURDAY

DAILY GOALS ACHIEVED

DAILY NUTRITIONAL INTAKE

Food/Beverages	Qty.	Calories	Fat	Carbs.	Protein	Fiber
DAILY TOTALS:						

DAILY EXERCISE

Activity	Hrs./Mins.	Cal. Burned
DAILY TOTALS:		

TIP OF THE DAY!

If having a cookout or barbecue, choose lean cuts of meat that have less fat or trim off excess fat before cooking.

DAILY NOTES, ACHIEVEMENTS

Obstacles, solutions, and thoughts on your progress.

_____
_____
_____
_____

DATE:

WEIGHT:

WATER INTAKE:
# of 8oz. glasses

☐ ☐ ☐ ☐
☐ ☐ ☐ ☐

ENERGY LEVEL:

☐ low
☐ medium
☐ high

DAILY # OF SERVINGS:

fruits

veggies

grains

meats & beans

milk & dairy

oils & sweets

VITAMINS & SUPPLEMENTS:

_____
_____
_____
_____
_____
_____
_____

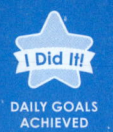

I Did It!

DAILY GOALS
ACHIEVED

WEEK
6

SUNDAY

DATE:

WEIGHT:

WATER INTAKE:
# of 8oz. glasses

☐ ☐ ☐ ☐
☐ ☐ ☐ ☐

ENERGY LEVEL:

☐ low
☐ medium
☐ high

DAILY # OF SERVINGS:

fruits

veggies

grains

meats & beans

milk & dairy

oils & sweets

VITAMINS & SUPPLEMENTS:

DAILY NUTRITIONAL INTAKE

Food/Beverages	Qty.	Calories	Fat	Carbs.	Protein	Fiber
DAILY TOTALS:						

DAILY EXERCISE

Activity	Hrs./Mins.	Cal. Burned
DAILY TOTALS:		

TIP OF THE DAY!

Fill up on low-density, high-volume foods, such as fruits, vegetables, soups and stews, cooked grains, lean meats, fish and lean poultry.

DAILY NOTES, ACHIEVEMENTS

Obstacles, solutions, and thoughts on your progress.

WEEKLY PROGRESS

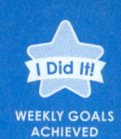

I Did It!

WEEKLY GOALS ACHIEVED

HIGHLIGHT OF THE WEEK

Your single-greatest moment of the week!

_____
_____
_____
_____

START WEIGHT:

END WEIGHT:

NUTRITIONAL INTAKE WRAP-UP

Did you meet your intake goals for the week? Why or why not?

_____
_____
_____
_____
_____
_____
_____

DAYS I TRACKED MY DIET:

- ☐ Mon.
- ☐ Tues.
- ☐ Wed.
- ☐ Thurs.
- ☐ Fri.
- ☐ Sat.
- ☐ Sun.

EXERCISE WRAP-UP

Did you meet your exercise goals for the week? Why or why not?

_____
_____
_____
_____
_____

DAYS I EXERCISED:

- ☐ Mon.
- ☐ Tues.
- ☐ Wed.
- ☐ Thurs.
- ☐ Fri.
- ☐ Sat.
- ☐ Sun.

GOALS FOR NEXT WEEK

Things to work on for next week.

_____
_____
_____
_____
_____
_____
_____

WEEKLY CALORIES BURNED:

WEEKLY ENERGY LEVEL:

- ☐ low
- ☐ medium
- ☐ high

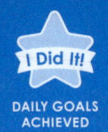
I Did It!

**DAILY GOALS
ACHIEVED**

WEEK 7 MONDAY

DATE:

WEIGHT:

WATER INTAKE:
# of 8oz. glasses

ENERGY LEVEL:
☐ low
☐ medium
☐ high

**DAILY # OF
SERVINGS:**

fruits

veggies

grains

meats &
beans

milk &
dairy

oils &
sweets

**VITAMINS &
SUPPLEMENTS:**

DAILY NUTRITIONAL INTAKE

Food/Beverages	Qty.	Calories	Fat	Carbs.	Protein	Fiber
DAILY TOTALS:						

DAILY EXERCISE

Activity	Hrs./Mins.	Cal. Burned
DAILY TOTALS:		

TIP OF THE DAY!

All oils are high in fat and calories, so be sure to go easy on the portions.

DAILY NOTES, ACHIEVEMENTS

Obstacles, solutions, and thoughts on your progress.

TUESDAY

DAILY GOALS ACHIEVED

DAILY NUTRITIONAL INTAKE

Food/Beverages	Qty.	Calories	Fat	Carbs.	Protein	Fiber
DAILY TOTALS:						

DAILY EXERCISE

Activity	Hrs./Mins.	Cal. Burned
DAILY TOTALS:		

TIP OF THE DAY!

Caffeine can give you that boost you need to wake up in the morning, but it can trick your body into thinking it is hungry when it is not.

DAILY NOTES, ACHIEVEMENTS

Obstacles, solutions, and thoughts on your progress.

DATE:

WEIGHT:

WATER INTAKE:
# of 8oz. glasses
☐ ☐ ☐ ☐
☐ ☐ ☐ ☐

ENERGY LEVEL:
☐ low
☐ medium
☐ high

DAILY # OF SERVINGS:

fruits

veggies

grains

meats & beans

milk & dairy

oils & sweets

VITAMINS & SUPPLEMENTS:

I Did It!

DAILY GOALS ACHIEVED

WEEK 7 WEDNESDAY

DATE:

WEIGHT:

WATER INTAKE:
# of 8oz. glasses

☐ ☐ ☐ ☐
☐ ☐ ☐ ☐

ENERGY LEVEL:

☐ low
☐ medium
☐ high

DAILY # OF SERVINGS:

fruits

veggies

grains

meats & beans

milk & dairy

oils & sweets

VITAMINS & SUPPLEMENTS:

DAILY NUTRITIONAL INTAKE

Food/Beverages	Qty.	Calories	Fat	Carbs.	Protein	Fiber
DAILY TOTALS:						

DAILY EXERCISE

Activity	Hrs./Mins.	Cal. Burned
DAILY TOTALS:		

TIP OF THE DAY!

Make the switch from sodas and coffee to water by gradually reducing the amount of caffeine you consume each day.

DAILY NOTES, ACHIEVEMENTS

Obstacles, solutions, and thoughts on your progress.

THURSDAY

DAILY GOALS ACHIEVED

DAILY NUTRITIONAL INTAKE

Food/Beverages	Qty.	Calories	Fat	Carbs.	Protein	Fiber
_____	_____					
_____	_____					
_____	_____					
_____	_____					
_____	_____					
_____	_____					
_____	_____					
_____	_____					
_____	_____					
_____	_____					
_____	_____					
_____	_____					
_____	_____					
_____	_____					
_____	_____					
_____	_____					
_____	_____					
_____	_____					
DAILY TOTALS:						

DATE:

WEIGHT:

WATER INTAKE:
# of 8oz. glasses

☐ ☐ ☐ ☐
☐ ☐ ☐ ☐

ENERGY LEVEL:
☐ low
☐ medium
☐ high

DAILY # OF SERVINGS:
- fruits
- veggies
- grains
- meats & beans
- milk & dairy
- oils & sweets

VITAMINS & SUPPLEMENTS:

_____
_____
_____
_____
_____

DAILY EXERCISE

Activity	Hrs./Mins.	Cal. Burned
_____	_____	
_____	_____	
_____	_____	
_____	_____	
_____	_____	
DAILY TOTALS:		

TIP OF THE DAY!

If you have diabetes, food allergies, or are a vegetarian, consult a dietetics professional on how you can safely lose weight.

DAILY NOTES, ACHIEVEMENTS

Obstacles, solutions, and thoughts on your progress.

_____
_____
_____

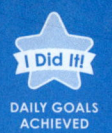

I Did It!

DAILY GOALS ACHIEVED

DATE:

WEIGHT:

WATER INTAKE:
# of 8oz. glasses

☐ ☐ ☐ ☐
☐ ☐ ☐ ☐

ENERGY LEVEL:

☐ low
☐ medium
☐ high

DAILY # OF SERVINGS:

fruits

veggies

grains

meats & beans

milk & dairy

oils & sweets

VITAMINS & SUPPLEMENTS:

DAILY NUTRITIONAL INTAKE

Food/Beverages	Qty.	Calories	Fat	Carbs.	Protein	Fiber
DAILY TOTALS:						

DAILY EXERCISE

Activity	Hrs./Mins.	Cal. Burned
DAILY TOTALS:		

TIP OF THE DAY!

Replacing full-sugar soda with water at mealtimes can help you lose around a pound a week.

DAILY NOTES, ACHIEVEMENTS

Obstacles, solutions, and thoughts on your progress.

SATURDAY

I Did It!

DAILY GOALS
ACHIEVED

DAILY NUTRITIONAL INTAKE

Food/Beverages	Qty.	Calories	Fat	Carbs.	Protein	Fiber
_____	___					
_____	___					
_____	___					
_____	___					
_____	___					
_____	___					
_____	___					
_____	___					
_____	___					
_____	___					
_____	___					
_____	___					
_____	___					
_____	___					
_____	___					
_____	___					
DAILY TOTALS:						

DATE:

WEIGHT:

WATER INTAKE:
# of 8oz. glasses
☐ ☐ ☐ ☐
☐ ☐ ☐ ☐

ENERGY LEVEL:
☐ low
☐ medium
☐ high

DAILY # OF SERVINGS:
fruits
veggies
grains
meats & beans
milk & dairy
oils & sweets

VITAMINS & SUPPLEMENTS:
_____
_____
_____
_____
_____
_____
_____
_____

DAILY EXERCISE

Activity	Hrs./Mins.	Cal. Burned
_____	_____	
_____	_____	
_____	_____	
_____	_____	
_____	_____	
DAILY TOTALS:		

TIP OF THE DAY!

If you are always on the go, traveling, or on vacation, pack healthy snacks like trail mix, dried fruits, nuts, or healthy crackers.

DAILY NOTES, ACHIEVEMENTS

Obstacles, solutions, and thoughts on your progress.

_____
_____
_____
_____

I Did It!
DAILY GOALS
ACHIEVED

SUNDAY

DATE:

WEIGHT:

WATER INTAKE:
# of 8oz. glasses
☐ ☐ ☐ ☐
☐ ☐ ☐ ☐

ENERGY LEVEL:
☐ low
☐ medium
☐ high

DAILY # OF SERVINGS:

fruits

veggies

grains

meats & beans

milk & dairy

oils & sweets

VITAMINS & SUPPLEMENTS:

DAILY NUTRITIONAL INTAKE							
Food/Beverages		Qty.	Calories	Fat	Carbs.	Protein	Fiber
DAILY TOTALS:							

DAILY EXERCISE		
Activity	Hrs./Mins.	Cal. Burned
DAILY TOTALS:		

TIP OF THE DAY!

Avoid processed foods, such as packaged snack foods and boxed meals, which contain high amounts of trans fats, artificial flavors, and preservatives.

DAILY NOTES, ACHIEVEMENTS
Obstacles, solutions, and thoughts on your progress.

WEEKLY PROGRESS

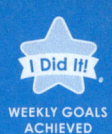

WEEKLY GOALS
ACHIEVED

HIGHLIGHT OF THE WEEK

Your single-greatest moment of the week!

_____

_____

_____

_____

START WEIGHT:

END WEIGHT:

NUTRITIONAL INTAKE WRAP-UP

Did you meet your intake goals for the week? Why or why not?

_____

_____

_____

_____

_____

_____

_____

DAYS I TRACKED MY DIET:

☐ Mon.
☐ Tues.
☐ Wed.
☐ Thurs.
☐ Fri.
☐ Sat.
☐ Sun.

EXERCISE WRAP-UP

Did you meet your exercise goals for the week? Why or why not?

_____

_____

_____

_____

_____

DAYS I EXERCISED:

☐ Mon.
☐ Tues.
☐ Wed.
☐ Thurs.
☐ Fri.
☐ Sat.
☐ Sun.

GOALS FOR NEXT WEEK

Things to work on for next week.

_____

_____

_____

_____

_____

_____

_____

_____

WEEKLY CALORIES BURNED:

WEEKLY ENERGY LEVEL:

☐ low
☐ medium
☐ high

I Did It!

DAILY GOALS ACHIEVED

WEEK
8

MONDAY

DATE:

WEIGHT:

WATER INTAKE:
# of 8oz. glasses

☐ ☐ ☐ ☐
☐ ☐ ☐ ☐

ENERGY LEVEL:

☐ low
☐ medium
☐ high

DAILY # OF SERVINGS:

fruits

veggies

grains

meats & beans

milk & dairy

oils & sweets

VITAMINS & SUPPLEMENTS:

DAILY NUTRITIONAL INTAKE						
Food/Beverages	Qty.	Calories	Fat	Carbs.	Protein	Fiber
DAILY TOTALS:						

DAILY EXERCISE		
Activity	Hrs./Mins.	Cal. Burned
DAILY TOTALS:		

TIP OF THE DAY!

Educate yourself on how to read a nutrition label. Understanding what is in the food you eat is an important step in your weight-loss program.

DAILY NOTES, ACHIEVEMENTS

Obstacles, solutions, and thoughts on your progress.

TUESDAY

DAILY GOALS ACHIEVED

DAILY NUTRITIONAL INTAKE

Food/Beverages	Qty.	Calories	Fat	Carbs.	Protein	Fiber
_____	____					
_____	____					
_____	____					
_____	____					
_____	____					
_____	____					
_____	____					
_____	____					
_____	____					
_____	____					
_____	____					
_____	____					
_____	____					
_____	____					
_____	____					
DAILY TOTALS:						

DAILY EXERCISE

Activity	Hrs./Mins.	Cal. Burned
_____	____	
_____	____	
_____	____	
_____	____	
_____	____	
DAILY TOTALS:		

TIP OF THE DAY!

Skip sugary juice in favor of eating whole fruits, or else make sure the juice you are drinking is 100 percent fruit juice.

DAILY NOTES, ACHIEVEMENTS

Obstacles, solutions, and thoughts on your progress.

_____

_____

_____

DATE:

WEIGHT:

WATER INTAKE:
# of 8oz. glasses

☐ ☐ ☐ ☐
☐ ☐ ☐ ☐

ENERGY LEVEL:

☐ low
☐ medium
☐ high

DAILY # OF SERVINGS:

fruits

veggies

grains

meats & beans

milk & dairy

oils & sweets

VITAMINS & SUPPLEMENTS:

_____

_____

_____

_____

_____

_____

_____

I Did It!

DAILY GOALS ACHIEVED

DATE:

WEIGHT:

WATER INTAKE:
# of 8oz. glasses

☐ ☐ ☐ ☐
☐ ☐ ☐ ☐

ENERGY LEVEL:

☐ low
☐ medium
☐ high

DAILY # OF SERVINGS:

fruits

veggies

grains

meats & beans

milk & dairy

oils & sweets

VITAMINS & SUPPLEMENTS:

DAILY NUTRITIONAL INTAKE

Food/Beverages	Qty.	Calories	Fat	Carbs.	Protein	Fiber
DAILY TOTALS:						

DAILY EXERCISE

Activity	Hrs./Mins.	Cal. Burned
DAILY TOTALS:		

TIP OF THE DAY!

Adopt a relaxation technique, such as yoga or deep breathing, to reduce your stress levels and lose weight.

DAILY NOTES, ACHIEVEMENTS

Obstacles, solutions, and thoughts on your progress.

THURSDAY

I Did It!

DAILY GOALS
ACHIEVED

DAILY NUTRITIONAL INTAKE

Food/Beverages	Qty.	Calories	Fat	Carbs.	Protein	Fiber
DAILY TOTALS:						

DAILY EXERCISE

Activity	Hrs./Mins.	Cal. Burned
DAILY TOTALS:		

TIP OF THE DAY!

Eating fish is a good way to increase the healthy fats in your diet, which can help reduce the risk of heart attacks.

DATE:

WEIGHT:

WATER INTAKE:

# of 8oz. glasses

☐ ☐ ☐ ☐
☐ ☐ ☐ ☐

ENERGY LEVEL:

☐ low
☐ medium
☐ high

DAILY # OF SERVINGS:

fruits

veggies

grains

meats & beans

milk & dairy

oils & sweets

VITAMINS & SUPPLEMENTS:

DAILY NOTES, ACHIEVEMENTS

Obstacles, solutions, and thoughts on your progress.

I Did It!
DAILY GOALS ACHIEVED

WEEK
8

FRIDAY

DATE:

WEIGHT:

WATER INTAKE:
# of 8oz. glasses

☐ ☐ ☐ ☐
☐ ☐ ☐ ☐

ENERGY LEVEL:
☐ low
☐ medium
☐ high

DAILY # OF SERVINGS:

fruits

veggies

grains

meats & beans

milk & dairy

oils & sweets

VITAMINS & SUPPLEMENTS:

DAILY NUTRITIONAL INTAKE						
Food/Beverages	Qty.	Calories	Fat	Carbs.	Protein	Fiber
DAILY TOTALS:						

DAILY EXERCISE			TIP OF THE DAY!
Activity	Hrs./Mins.	Cal. Burned	

TIP OF THE DAY!

Choose carbs wisely. Eat a 100-calorie apple versus eating a 100-calorie serving of chips.

DAILY TOTALS:

DAILY NOTES, ACHIEVEMENTS
Obstacles, solutions, and thoughts on your progress.

SATURDAY

I Did It!

DAILY GOALS
ACHIEVED

DAILY NUTRITIONAL INTAKE

Food/Beverages	Qty.	Calories	Fat	Carbs.	Protein	Fiber
DAILY TOTALS:						

DAILY EXERCISE

Activity	Hrs./Mins.	Cal. Burned
DAILY TOTALS:		

TIP OF THE DAY!

Be sure to get enough calcium in your diet, through dairy, green leafy vegetables, or supplements.

DAILY NOTES, ACHIEVEMENTS

Obstacles, solutions, and thoughts on your progress.

DATE:

WEIGHT:

WATER INTAKE:
# of 8oz. glasses

☐ ☐ ☐ ☐
☐ ☐ ☐ ☐

ENERGY LEVEL:

☐ low
☐ medium
☐ high

DAILY # OF SERVINGS:

fruits

veggies

grains

meats & beans

milk & dairy

oils & sweets

VITAMINS & SUPPLEMENTS:

I Did It!

DAILY GOALS ACHIEVED

WEEK
8

SUNDAY

DATE:

WEIGHT:

WATER INTAKE:
# of 8oz. glasses

☐ ☐ ☐ ☐
☐ ☐ ☐ ☐

ENERGY LEVEL:
☐ low
☐ medium
☐ high

DAILY # OF SERVINGS:

fruits

veggies

grains

meats & beans

milk & dairy

oils & sweets

VITAMINS & SUPPLEMENTS:

DAILY NUTRITIONAL INTAKE						
Food/Beverages	Qty.	Calories	Fat	Carbs.	Protein	Fiber
DAILY TOTALS:						

DAILY EXERCISE		
Activity	Hrs./Mins.	Cal. Burned
DAILY TOTALS:		

TIP OF THE DAY!

Having a small snack between meals can help you control your appetite, provides you with energy, and keeps your metabolism active.

DAILY NOTES, ACHIEVEMENTS

Obstacles, solutions, and thoughts on your progress.

WEEKLY PROGRESS

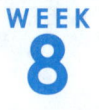
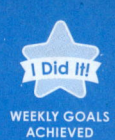

I Did It!

WEEKLY GOALS
ACHIEVED

HIGHLIGHT OF THE WEEK

Your single-greatest moment of the week!

_____

_____

_____

_____

START WEIGHT:

END WEIGHT:

NUTRITIONAL INTAKE WRAP-UP

Did you meet your intake goals for the week? Why or why not?

_____

_____

_____

_____

_____

_____

_____

DAYS I TRACKED MY DIET:

- ☐ Mon.
- ☐ Tues.
- ☐ Wed.
- ☐ Thurs.
- ☐ Fri.
- ☐ Sat.
- ☐ Sun.

EXERCISE WRAP-UP

Did you meet your exercise goals for the week? Why or why not?

_____

_____

_____

_____

_____

DAYS I EXERCISED:

- ☐ Mon.
- ☐ Tues.
- ☐ Wed.
- ☐ Thurs.
- ☐ Fri.
- ☐ Sat.
- ☐ Sun.

GOALS FOR NEXT WEEK

Things to work on for next week.

_____

_____

_____

_____

_____

_____

_____

_____

WEEKLY CALORIES BURNED:

WEEKLY ENERGY LEVEL:

- ☐ low
- ☐ medium
- ☐ high

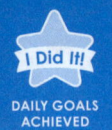

I Did It!

DAILY GOALS
ACHIEVED

WEEK
9

MONDAY

DATE:

WEIGHT:

WATER INTAKE:
# of 8oz. glasses

☐ ☐ ☐ ☐
☐ ☐ ☐ ☐

ENERGY LEVEL:
☐ low
☐ medium
☐ high

DAILY # OF
SERVINGS:

fruits

veggies

grains

meats &
beans

milk &
dairy

oils &
sweets

VITAMINS &
SUPPLEMENTS:

DAILY NUTRITIONAL INTAKE

Food/Beverages	Qty.	Calories	Fat	Carbs.	Protein	Fiber
DAILY TOTALS:						

DAILY EXERCISE

Activity	Hrs./Mins.	Cal. Burned
DAILY TOTALS:		

TIP OF THE DAY!

Body mass index (BMI)
is a good indicator of
whether or not you
are at a healthy
weight.

DAILY NOTES, ACHIEVEMENTS

Obstacles, solutions, and thoughts on your progress.

TUESDAY

DAILY GOALS ACHIEVED

DAILY NUTRITIONAL INTAKE

Food/Beverages	Qty.	Calories	Fat	Carbs.	Protein	Fiber
DAILY TOTALS:						

DAILY EXERCISE

Activity	Hrs./Mins.	Cal. Burned
DAILY TOTALS:		

TIP OF THE DAY!

Try to prepare meals in advance if you know you are going to be busy and unable to cook a proper meal.

DAILY NOTES, ACHIEVEMENTS

Obstacles, solutions, and thoughts on your progress.

DATE:

WEIGHT:

WATER INTAKE:
# of 8oz. glasses

☐ ☐ ☐ ☐
☐ ☐ ☐ ☐

ENERGY LEVEL:

☐ low

☐ medium

☐ high

DAILY # OF SERVINGS:

fruits

veggies

grains

meats & beans

milk & dairy

oils & sweets

VITAMINS & SUPPLEMENTS:

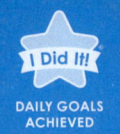

I Did It!
DAILY GOALS
ACHIEVED

DATE:

WEIGHT:

WATER INTAKE:
# of 8oz. glasses

☐ ☐ ☐ ☐
☐ ☐ ☐ ☐

ENERGY LEVEL:
☐ low
☐ medium
☐ high

DAILY # OF SERVINGS:

fruits

veggies

grains

meats & beans

milk & dairy

oils & sweets

VITAMINS & SUPPLEMENTS:

DAILY NUTRITIONAL INTAKE

Food/Beverages	Qty.	Calories	Fat	Carbs.	Protein	Fiber
DAILY TOTALS:						

DAILY EXERCISE

Activity	Hrs./Mins.	Cal. Burned
DAILY TOTALS:		

TIP OF THE DAY!

Adopt a lifestyle that includes all foods in moderation, healthy alternatives to foods high in fat and calories, and daily activities.

DAILY NOTES, ACHIEVEMENTS

Obstacles, solutions, and thoughts on your progress.

THURSDAY

I Did It!

DAILY GOALS
ACHIEVED

DAILY NUTRITIONAL INTAKE

Food/Beverages	Qty.	Calories	Fat	Carbs.	Protein	Fiber
DAILY TOTALS:						

DATE:

WEIGHT:

WATER INTAKE:
# of 8oz. glasses
☐ ☐ ☐ ☐
☐ ☐ ☐ ☐

ENERGY LEVEL:
☐ low
☐ medium
☐ high

DAILY # OF SERVINGS:

fruits

veggies

grains

meats & beans

milk & dairy

oils & sweets

VITAMINS & SUPPLEMENTS:

DAILY EXERCISE

Activity	Hrs./Mins.	Cal. Burned
DAILY TOTALS:		

TIP OF THE DAY!

Studies have shown that adding more plant foods to your diet is a good way to lower your LDL or "bad" cholesterol levels.

DAILY NOTES, ACHIEVEMENTS

Obstacles, solutions, and thoughts on your progress.

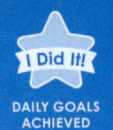

I Did It!

DAILY GOALS
ACHIEVED

WEEK 9 FRIDAY

DATE:

WEIGHT:

WATER INTAKE:

# of 8oz. glasses

☐ ☐ ☐ ☐
☐ ☐ ☐ ☐

ENERGY LEVEL:

☐ low
☐ medium
☐ high

DAILY # OF SERVINGS:

fruits

veggies

grains

meats & beans

milk & dairy

oils & sweets

VITAMINS & SUPPLEMENTS:

DAILY NUTRITIONAL INTAKE

Food/Beverages	Qty.	Calories	Fat	Carbs.	Protein	Fiber
DAILY TOTALS:						

DAILY EXERCISE

Activity	Hrs./Mins.	Cal. Burned
DAILY TOTALS:		

TIP OF THE DAY!

Add more plant foods to your diet by including oats, barley, dried beans, oranges, apples, and nuts.

DAILY NOTES, ACHIEVEMENTS

Obstacles, solutions, and thoughts on your progress.

SATURDAY

I Did It!

DAILY GOALS
ACHIEVED

DAILY NUTRITIONAL INTAKE

Food/Beverages	Qty.	Calories	Fat	Carbs.	Protein	Fiber
DAILY TOTALS:						

DATE:

WEIGHT:

WATER INTAKE:
of 8oz. glasses

☐ ☐ ☐ ☐
☐ ☐ ☐ ☐

ENERGY LEVEL:

☐ low
☐ medium
☐ high

DAILY # OF SERVINGS:

fruits

veggies

grains

meats & beans

milk & dairy

oils & sweets

VITAMINS & SUPPLEMENTS:

DAILY EXERCISE

Activity	Hrs./Mins.	Cal. Burned
DAILY TOTALS:		

TIP OF THE DAY!

Enriched foods have nutrients added to them that were lost during food processing. Fortified foods have nutrients added that were not originally present.

DAILY NOTES, ACHIEVEMENTS

Obstacles, solutions, and thoughts on your progress.

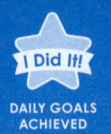

I Did It!

DAILY GOALS
ACHIEVED

SUNDAY

DATE:

WEIGHT:

WATER INTAKE:
# of 8oz. glasses

☐ ☐ ☐ ☐
☐ ☐ ☐ ☐

ENERGY LEVEL:

☐ low
☐ medium
☐ high

**DAILY # OF
SERVINGS:**

fruits

veggies

grains

meats &
beans

milk &
dairy

oils &
sweets

**VITAMINS &
SUPPLEMENTS:**

_____

_____

_____

_____

_____

DAILY NUTRITIONAL INTAKE

Food/Beverages	Qty.	Calories	Fat	Carbs.	Protein	Fiber
_____	_____					
_____	_____					
_____	_____					
_____	_____					
_____	_____					
_____	_____					
_____	_____					
_____	_____					
_____	_____					
_____	_____					
_____	_____					
_____	_____					
_____	_____					
_____	_____					
_____	_____					

DAILY TOTALS:

DAILY EXERCISE

Activity	Hrs./Mins.	Cal. Burned
_____	_____	
_____	_____	
_____	_____	
_____	_____	
_____	_____	

DAILY TOTALS:

TIP OF THE DAY!

Fruits and vegetables
have a high fiber and
water content, which
means they fill you up
and keep you full
longer.

DAILY NOTES, ACHIEVEMENTS

Obstacles, solutions, and thoughts on your progress.

_____

_____

_____

WEEKLY PROGRESS

 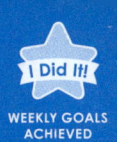

I Did It!
WEEKLY GOALS
ACHIEVED

HIGHLIGHT OF THE WEEK
Your single-greatest moment of the week!

_____

_____

_____

_____

NUTRITIONAL INTAKE WRAP-UP
Did you meet your intake goals for the week? Why or why not?

_____

_____

_____

_____

_____

_____

EXERCISE WRAP-UP
Did you meet your exercise goals for the week? Why or why not?

_____

_____

_____

_____

GOALS FOR NEXT WEEK
Things to work on for next week.

_____

_____

_____

_____

_____

_____

START WEIGHT:

END WEIGHT:

DAYS I TRACKED MY DIET:
- [ ] Mon.
- [ ] Tues.
- [ ] Wed.
- [ ] Thurs.
- [ ] Fri.
- [ ] Sat.
- [ ] Sun.

DAYS I EXERCISED:
- [ ] Mon.
- [ ] Tues.
- [ ] Wed.
- [ ] Thurs.
- [ ] Fri.
- [ ] Sat.
- [ ] Sun.

WEEKLY CALORIES BURNED:

WEEKLY ENERGY LEVEL:
- [ ] low
- [ ] medium
- [ ] high

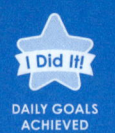

I Did It!
DAILY GOALS
ACHIEVED

MONDAY

DATE:

WEIGHT:

WATER INTAKE:
# of 8oz. glasses
☐ ☐ ☐ ☐
☐ ☐ ☐ ☐

ENERGY LEVEL:
☐ low
☐ medium
☐ high

DAILY # OF SERVINGS:

fruits

veggies

grains

meats & beans

milk & dairy

oils & sweets

VITAMINS & SUPPLEMENTS:

DAILY NUTRITIONAL INTAKE						
Food/Beverages	Qty.	Calories	Fat	Carbs.	Protein	Fiber
DAILY TOTALS:						

DAILY EXERCISE		
Activity	Hrs./Mins.	Cal. Burned
DAILY TOTALS:		

TIP OF THE DAY!

Eating 5 small meals a day is a good way to control your eating habits and portion sizes.

DAILY NOTES, ACHIEVEMENTS

Obstacles, solutions, and thoughts on your progress.

TUESDAY

I Did It!

DAILY GOALS ACHIEVED

DAILY NUTRITIONAL INTAKE

Food/Beverages	Qty.	Calories	Fat	Carbs.	Protein	Fiber
DAILY TOTALS:						

DATE:

WEIGHT:

WATER INTAKE:
# of 8oz. glasses

☐ ☐ ☐ ☐
☐ ☐ ☐ ☐

ENERGY LEVEL:

☐ low
☐ medium
☐ high

DAILY # OF SERVINGS:

fruits

veggies

grains

meats & beans

milk & dairy

oils & sweets

VITAMINS & SUPPLEMENTS:

DAILY EXERCISE

Activity	Hrs./Mins.	Cal. Burned
DAILY TOTALS:		

TIP OF THE DAY!

Ginger, cinnamon, nutmeg, and vanilla are all good additions to food in order to curb a sweet tooth.

DAILY NOTES, ACHIEVEMENTS

Obstacles, solutions, and thoughts on your progress.

I Did It!

DAILY GOALS
ACHIEVED

DATE:

WEIGHT:

WATER INTAKE:
# of 8oz. glasses

☐ ☐ ☐ ☐
☐ ☐ ☐ ☐

ENERGY LEVEL:

☐ low
☐ medium
☐ high

DAILY # OF SERVINGS:

fruits

veggies

grains

meats & beans

milk & dairy

oils & sweets

VITAMINS & SUPPLEMENTS:

DAILY NUTRITIONAL INTAKE

Food/Beverages	Qty.	Calories	Fat	Carbs.	Protein	Fiber
DAILY TOTALS:						

DAILY EXERCISE

Activity	Hrs./Mins.	Cal. Burned
DAILY TOTALS:		

TIP OF THE DAY!

Just because a product claims that it is "low fat," "fat-free," "sugar-free," or "low carb" does not necessarily mean they will help you lose weight.

DAILY NOTES, ACHIEVEMENTS

Obstacles, solutions, and thoughts on your progress.

THURSDAY

 DAILY GOALS ACHIEVED

DAILY NUTRITIONAL INTAKE

Food/Beverages	Qty.	Calories	Fat	Carbs.	Protein	Fiber
DAILY TOTALS:						

DAILY EXERCISE

Activity	Hrs./Mins.	Cal. Burned
DAILY TOTALS:		

TIP OF THE DAY!

If you're looking for a quick, healthy afternoon snack, try munching on slices of fruit, low-fat popcorn, mixed nuts, or trail mix.

DAILY NOTES, ACHIEVEMENTS

Obstacles, solutions, and thoughts on your progress.

_____
_____
_____

DATE:

WEIGHT:

WATER INTAKE:
# of 8oz. glasses

☐ ☐ ☐ ☐
☐ ☐ ☐ ☐

ENERGY LEVEL:

☐ low
☐ medium
☐ high

DAILY # OF SERVINGS:

fruits

veggies

grains

meats & beans

milk & dairy

oils & sweets

VITAMINS & SUPPLEMENTS:

_____

_____

_____

_____

_____

_____

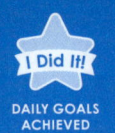

I Did It!

DAILY GOALS
ACHIEVED

DATE:

WEIGHT:

WATER INTAKE:
# of 8oz. glasses

☐ ☐ ☐ ☐
☐ ☐ ☐ ☐

ENERGY LEVEL:
☐ low
☐ medium
☐ high

DAILY # OF SERVINGS:

fruits

veggies

grains

meats & beans

milk & dairy

oils & sweets

VITAMINS & SUPPLEMENTS:

DAILY NUTRITIONAL INTAKE

Food/Beverages	Qty.	Calories	Fat	Carbs.	Protein	Fiber
DAILY TOTALS:						

DAILY EXERCISE

Activity	Hrs./Mins.	Cal. Burned
DAILY TOTALS:		

TIP OF THE DAY!

Make your meals seem like more food
by serving them on smaller plates.

DAILY NOTES, ACHIEVEMENTS

Obstacles, solutions, and thoughts on your progress.

SATURDAY

I Did It!

DAILY GOALS
ACHIEVED

DAILY NUTRITIONAL INTAKE

Food/Beverages	Qty.	Calories	Fat	Carbs.	Protein	Fiber
_____	_____					
_____	_____					
_____	_____					
_____	_____					
_____	_____					
_____	_____					
_____	_____					
_____	_____					
_____	_____					
_____	_____					
_____	_____					
_____	_____					
_____	_____					
_____	_____					
_____	_____					
_____	_____					
DAILY TOTALS:						

DATE:

WEIGHT:

WATER INTAKE:
# of 8oz. glasses
☐ ☐ ☐ ☐
☐ ☐ ☐ ☐

ENERGY LEVEL:
☐ low
☐ medium
☐ high

DAILY # OF
SERVINGS:

____ fruits

____ veggies

____ grains

____ meats &
beans

____ milk &
dairy

____ oils &
sweets

VITAMINS &
SUPPLEMENTS:

_____

_____

_____

_____

_____

_____

DAILY EXERCISE

Activity	Hrs./Mins.	Cal. Burned
_____	_____	
_____	_____	
_____	_____	
_____	_____	
_____	_____	
DAILY TOTALS:		

TIP OF THE DAY!

Eat more slowly.
When you eat at a
slower pace, you give
yourself more time to
recognize when you
are full.

DAILY NOTES, ACHIEVEMENTS

Obstacles, solutions, and thoughts on your progress.

_____

_____

_____

_____

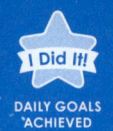

I Did It!

DAILY GOALS
*ACHIEVED

DATE:

WEIGHT:

WATER INTAKE:
# of 8oz. glasses

☐ ☐ ☐ ☐
☐ ☐ ☐ ☐

ENERGY LEVEL:
☐ low
☐ medium
☐ high

DAILY # OF SERVINGS:

fruits

veggies

grains

meats & beans

milk & dairy

oils & sweets

VITAMINS & SUPPLEMENTS:

DAILY NUTRITIONAL INTAKE

Food/Beverages	Qty.	Calories	Fat	Carbs.	Protein	Fiber
DAILY TOTALS:						

DAILY EXERCISE

Activity	Hrs./Mins.	Cal. Burned
DAILY TOTALS:		

TIP OF THE DAY!

Heat up your food. Foods served hot can be more satiating so you are likely to eat less.

DAILY NOTES, ACHIEVEMENTS

Obstacles, solutions, and thoughts on your progress.

WEEKLY PROGRESS

WEEK 10

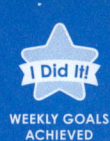

I Did It!

WEEKLY GOALS ACHIEVED

HIGHLIGHT OF THE WEEK

Your single-greatest moment of the week!

_____
_____
_____
_____
_____

START WEIGHT:

END WEIGHT:

NUTRITIONAL INTAKE WRAP-UP

Did you meet your intake goals for the week? Why or why not?

_____
_____
_____
_____
_____
_____
_____

DAYS I TRACKED MY DIET:

☐ Mon.
☐ Tues.
☐ Wed.
☐ Thurs.
☐ Fri.
☐ Sat.
☐ Sun.

EXERCISE WRAP-UP

Did you meet your exercise goals for the week? Why or why not?

_____
_____
_____
_____

DAYS I EXERCISED:

☐ Mon.
☐ Tues.
☐ Wed.
☐ Thurs.
☐ Fri.
☐ Sat.
☐ Sun.

GOALS FOR NEXT WEEK

Things to work on for next week.

_____
_____
_____
_____
_____
_____
_____
_____

WEEKLY CALORIES BURNED:

WEEKLY ENERGY LEVEL:

☐ low
☐ medium
☐ high

MONTHLY

DATE:

START WEIGHT:

END WEIGHT:

BODY FAT %:

MEASUREMENTS:

chest

biceps

waist

hips

thighs

NOTES:

PHOTO OF THE MONTH

Photo comments.

tape your photo here

PROGRESS

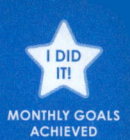

I DID IT!

MONTHLY GOALS ACHIEVED

HIGHLIGHT OF THE MONTH

Your single-greatest moment of the month!

_____

_____

_____

_____

_____

NUTRITIONAL INTAKE WRAP-UP

Did you meet your intake goals for the month? Why or why not?

_____

_____

_____

_____

_____

_____

_____

EXERCISE WRAP-UP

Did you meet your exercise goals for the month? Why or why not?

_____

_____

_____

_____

_____

GOALS FOR NEXT MONTH

Things to work on for next month.

_____

_____

_____

_____

_____

_____

_____

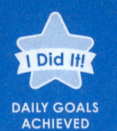
I Did It!
DAILY GOALS
ACHIEVED

WEEK 11
MONDAY

DATE:

WEIGHT:

WATER INTAKE:
# of 8oz. glasses

☐ ☐ ☐ ☐
☐ ☐ ☐ ☐

ENERGY LEVEL:
☐ low
☐ medium
☐ high

DAILY # OF SERVINGS:

fruits

veggies

grains

meats & beans

milk & dairy

oils & sweets

VITAMINS & SUPPLEMENTS:

DAILY NUTRITIONAL INTAKE

Food/Beverages	Qty.	Calories	Fat	Carbs.	Protein	Fiber
DAILY TOTALS:						

DAILY EXERCISE

Activity	Hrs./Mins.	Cal. Burned
DAILY TOTALS:		

TIP OF THE DAY!

When eating, try to savor each bite of food. Putting your fork down between bites can help you control your portion sizes so you don't overeat.

DAILY NOTES, ACHIEVEMENTS

Obstacles, solutions, and thoughts on your progress.

TUESDAY

I Did It!

DAILY GOALS
ACHIEVED

DAILY NUTRITIONAL INTAKE

Food/Beverages	Qty.	Calories	Fat	Carbs.	Protein	Fiber
DAILY TOTALS:						

DATE:

WEIGHT:

WATER INTAKE:
# of 8oz. glasses

☐ ☐ ☐ ☐
☐ ☐ ☐ ☐

ENERGY LEVEL:

☐ low
☐ medium
☐ high

DAILY # OF SERVINGS:

fruits

veggies

grains

meats & beans

milk & dairy

oils & sweets

VITAMINS & SUPPLEMENTS:

DAILY EXERCISE

Activity	Hrs./Mins.	Cal. Burned
DAILY TOTALS:		

TIP OF THE DAY!

Men and women who eat breakfast in the mornings are far less likely to become obese than those who skip the most important meal of the day.

DAILY NOTES, ACHIEVEMENTS

Obstacles, solutions, and thoughts on your progress.

I Did It!
DAILY GOALS
ACHIEVED

DATE:

WEIGHT:

WATER INTAKE:
# of 8oz. glasses

☐ ☐ ☐ ☐
☐ ☐ ☐ ☐

ENERGY LEVEL:

☐ low
☐ medium
☐ high

DAILY # OF SERVINGS:

fruits

veggies

grains

meats & beans

milk & dairy

oils & sweets

VITAMINS & SUPPLEMENTS:

DAILY NUTRITIONAL INTAKE

Food/Beverages	Qty.	Calories	Fat	Carbs.	Protein	Fiber
DAILY TOTALS:						

DAILY EXERCISE

Activity	Hrs./Mins.	Cal. Burned
DAILY TOTALS:		

TIP OF THE DAY!

Switch to taller, narrow glasses to keep from drinking extra calories. People tend to think that a tall glass contains more liquid than a short, wide tumbler.

DAILY NOTES, ACHIEVEMENTS

Obstacles, solutions, and thoughts on your progress.

THURSDAY

I Did It!

DAILY GOALS
ACHIEVED

DAILY NUTRITIONAL INTAKE

Food/Beverages	Qty.	Calories	Fat	Carbs.	Protein	Fiber
DAILY TOTALS:						

DAILY EXERCISE

Activity	Hrs./Mins.	Cal. Burned
DAILY TOTALS:		

TIP OF THE DAY!

Try not to go to the grocery store when you are hungry. It can lead to buying more food than you need.

DAILY NOTES, ACHIEVEMENTS

Obstacles, solutions, and thoughts on your progress.

_____

_____

_____

_____

DATE:

WEIGHT:

WATER INTAKE:

# of 8oz. glasses

☐ ☐ ☐ ☐
☐ ☐ ☐ ☐

ENERGY LEVEL:

☐ low

☐ medium

☐ high

DAILY # OF SERVINGS:

fruits

veggies

grains

meats & beans

milk & dairy

oils & sweets

VITAMINS & SUPPLEMENTS:

_____

_____

_____

_____

_____

_____

_____

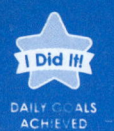

I Did It!

DAILY GOALS
ACHIEVED

DATE:

WEIGHT:

WATER INTAKE:
# of 8oz. glasses

☐ ☐ ☐ ☐
☐ ☐ ☐ ☐

ENERGY LEVEL:
☐ low
☐ medium
☐ high

DAILY # OF SERVINGS:

fruits

veggies

grains

meats & beans

milk & dairy

oils & sweets

VITAMINS & SUPPLEMENTS:

DAILY NUTRITIONAL INTAKE

Food/Beverages	Qty.	Calories	Fat	Carbs.	Protein	Fiber
DAILY TOTALS:						

DAILY EXERCISE

Activity	Hrs./Mins.	Cal. Burned
DAILY TOTALS:		

TIP OF THE DAY!

Instead of fixating on all the "bad stuff," write down all of the physical qualities you like about yourself and the good things you have done for your body.

DAILY NOTES, ACHIEVEMENTS

Obstacles, solutions, and thoughts on your progress.

SATURDAY

I Did It!

DAILY GOALS ACHIEVED.

DAILY NUTRITIONAL INTAKE

Food/Beverages	Qty.	Calories	Fat	Carbs.	Protein	Fiber
DAILY TOTALS:						

DAILY EXERCISE

Activity	Hrs./Mins.	Cal. Burned
DAILY TOTALS:		

TIP OF THE DAY!

Nuts are a great snack item. They are high in monounsaturated fats, protein, and carbohydrates, as well as vitamins and minerals.

DAILY NOTES, ACHIEVEMENTS

Obstacles, solutions, and thoughts on your progress.

DATE:

WEIGHT:

WATER INTAKE:
# of 8oz. glasses

☐ ☐ ☐ ☐
☐ ☐ ☐ ☐

ENERGY LEVEL:
☐ low
☐ medium
☐ high

DAILY # OF SERVINGS:

fruits

veggies

grains

meats & beans

milk & dairy

oils & sweets

VITAMINS & SUPPLEMENTS:

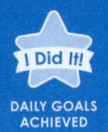

I Did It!

DAILY GOALS
ACHIEVED

DATE:

WEIGHT:

WATER INTAKE:
# of 8oz. glasses

☐ ☐ ☐ ☐
☐ ☐ ☐ ☐

ENERGY LEVEL:

☐ low
☐ medium
☐ high

DAILY # OF SERVINGS:

fruits

veggies

grains

meats & beans

milk & dairy

oils & sweets

VITAMINS & SUPPLEMENTS:

DAILY NUTRITIONAL INTAKE

Food/Beverages	Qty.	Calories	Fat	Carbs.	Protein	Fiber
DAILY TOTALS:						

DAILY EXERCISE

Activity	Hrs./Mins.	Cal. Burned
DAILY TOTALS:		

TIP OF THE DAY!

Snacking on nuts can lead to eating less and losing weight. However, because nuts are high in calories, just be sure to eat only small servings at a time.

DAILY NOTES, ACHIEVEMENTS

Obstacles, solutions, and thoughts on your progress.

WEEKLY PROGRESS

WEEK 11

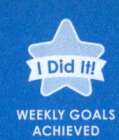

I Did It!
WEEKLY GOALS
ACHIEVED

HIGHLIGHT OF THE WEEK

Your single-greatest moment of the week!

_____
_____
_____
_____

START WEIGHT:

END WEIGHT:

NUTRITIONAL INTAKE WRAP-UP

Did you meet your intake goals for the week? Why or why not?

_____
_____
_____
_____
_____
_____
_____

DAYS I TRACKED MY DIET:

☐ Mon.
☐ Tues.
☐ Wed.
☐ Thurs.
☐ Fri.
☐ Sat.
☐ Sun.

EXERCISE WRAP-UP

Did you meet your exercise goals for the week? Why or why not?

_____
_____
_____
_____
_____

DAYS I EXERCISED:

☐ Mon.
☐ Tues.
☐ Wed.
☐ Thurs.
☐ Fri.
☐ Sat.
☐ Sun.

GOALS FOR NEXT WEEK

Things to work on for next week.

_____
_____
_____
_____
_____
_____
_____

WEEKLY CALORIES BURNED:

WEEKLY ENERGY LEVEL:

☐ low
☐ medium
☐ high

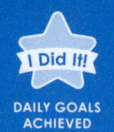

I Did It!

DAILY GOALS ACHIEVED

DATE:

WEIGHT:

WATER INTAKE:
# of 8oz. glasses

☐ ☐ ☐ ☐
☐ ☐ ☐ ☐

ENERGY LEVEL:

☐ low
☐ medium
☐ high

DAILY # OF SERVINGS:

fruits

veggies

grains

meats & beans

milk & dairy

oils & sweets

VITAMINS & SUPPLEMENTS:

DAILY NUTRITIONAL INTAKE

Food/Beverages	Qty.	Calories	Fat	Carbs.	Protein	Fiber
DAILY TOTALS:						

DAILY EXERCISE

Activity	Hrs./Mins.	Cal. Burned
DAILY TOTALS:		

TIP OF THE DAY!

Drinking 1 glass of red wine at night may help improve your HDL, or "good" cholesterol levels while reducing your LDL, or "bad" cholesterol levels.

DAILY NOTES, ACHIEVEMENTS

Obstacles, solutions, and thoughts on your progress.

TUESDAY

I Did It!
DAILY GOALS
ACHIEVED

DAILY NUTRITIONAL INTAKE

Food/Beverages	Qty.	Calories	Fat	Carbs.	Protein	Fiber
DAILY TOTALS:						

DAILY EXERCISE

Activity	Hrs./Mins.	Cal. Burned
DAILY TOTALS:		

TIP OF THE DAY!

Try grilling, sautéing, or baking your food instead of frying it. The way you prepare your food has a big influence on how good it is for you.

DAILY NOTES, ACHIEVEMENTS

Obstacles, solutions, and thoughts on your progress.

DATE:

WEIGHT:

WATER INTAKE:
# of 8oz. glasses
☐ ☐ ☐ ☐
☐ ☐ ☐ ☐

ENERGY LEVEL:
☐ low
☐ medium
☐ high

DAILY # OF SERVINGS:

fruits

veggies

grains

meats & beans

milk & dairy

oils & sweets

VITAMINS & SUPPLEMENTS:

I Did It!

DAILY GOALS
ACHIEVED

DATE:

WEIGHT:

WATER INTAKE:
# of 8oz. glasses

☐ ☐ ☐ ☐
☐ ☐ ☐ ☐

ENERGY LEVEL:
☐ low
☐ medium
☐ high

DAILY # OF SERVINGS:

fruits

veggies

grains

meats & beans

milk & dairy

oils & sweets

VITAMINS & SUPPLEMENTS:

DAILY NUTRITIONAL INTAKE

Food/Beverages	Qty.	Calories	Fat	Carbs.	Protein	Fiber
DAILY TOTALS:						

DAILY EXERCISE

Activity	Hrs./Mins.	Cal. Burned
DAILY TOTALS:		

TIP OF THE DAY!

Schedule an event that you would like to lose weight for, such as your birthday, a vacation, or high school reunion.

DAILY NOTES, ACHIEVEMENTS

Obstacles, solutions, and thoughts on your progress.

THURSDAY

I Did It!

DAILY GOALS
ACHIEVED

DAILY NUTRITIONAL INTAKE

Food/Beverages	Qty.	Calories	Fat	Carbs.	Protein	Fiber
_____	_____					
_____	_____					
_____	_____					
_____	_____					
_____	_____					
_____	_____					
_____	_____					
_____	_____					
_____	_____					
_____	_____					
_____	_____					
_____	_____					
_____	_____					
_____	_____					
_____	_____					
DAILY TOTALS:						

DATE:

WEIGHT:

WATER INTAKE:
# of 8oz. glasses

☐ ☐ ☐ ☐
☐ ☐ ☐ ☐

ENERGY LEVEL:

☐ low
☐ medium
☐ high

DAILY # OF SERVINGS:

fruits

veggies

grains

meats & beans

milk & dairy

oils & sweets

DAILY EXERCISE

Activity	Hrs./Mins.	Cal. Burned
_____	_____	
_____	_____	
_____	_____	
_____	_____	
DAILY TOTALS:		

TIP OF THE DAY!

Remember that small measurable steps toward weight loss are often the most gratifying.

VITAMINS & SUPPLEMENTS:

_____
_____
_____
_____
_____
_____
_____

DAILY NOTES, ACHIEVEMENTS

Obstacles, solutions, and thoughts on your progress.

_____
_____
_____

I Did It!
DAILY GOALS
ACHIEVED

WEEK
12

FRIDAY

DATE:

WEIGHT:

WATER INTAKE:
# of 8oz. glasses

☐ ☐ ☐ ☐
☐ ☐ ☐ ☐

ENERGY LEVEL:
☐ low
☐ medium
☐ high

DAILY # OF SERVINGS:

fruits

veggies

grains

meats & beans

milk & dairy

oils & sweets

VITAMINS & SUPPLEMENTS:

DAILY NUTRITIONAL INTAKE

Food/Beverages	Qty.	Calories	Fat	Carbs.	Protein	Fiber
DAILY TOTALS:						

DAILY EXERCISE

Activity	Hrs./Mins.	Cal. Burned
DAILY TOTALS:		

TIP OF THE DAY!

Stay motivated by documenting changes to your weight, body size, energy and mood on a weekly and monthly basis.

DAILY NOTES, ACHIEVEMENTS

Obstacles, solutions, and thoughts on your progress.

SATURDAY

DAILY GOALS
ACHIEVED

DAILY NUTRITIONAL INTAKE

Food/Beverages	Qty.	Calories	Fat	Carbs.	Protein	Fiber
_____	____					
_____	____					
_____	____					
_____	____					
_____	____					
_____	____					
_____	____					
_____	____					
_____	____					
_____	____					
_____	____					
_____	____					
_____	____					
_____	____					
_____	____					
_____	____					
DAILY TOTALS:						

DATE:

WEIGHT:

WATER INTAKE:
# of 8oz. glasses
☐ ☐ ☐ ☐
☐ ☐ ☐ ☐

ENERGY LEVEL:
☐ low
☐ medium
☐ high

DAILY # OF SERVINGS:

fruits

veggies

grains

meats & beans

milk & dairy

oils & sweets

DAILY EXERCISE

Activity	Hrs./Mins.	Cal. Burned
_____	_____	
_____	_____	
_____	_____	
_____	_____	
_____	_____	
DAILY TOTALS:		

TIP OF THE DAY!

If you feel a craving coming on, try to distract yourself by taking a walk or calling a friend.

VITAMINS & SUPPLEMENTS:

_____

_____

_____

_____

_____

_____

_____

DAILY NOTES, ACHIEVEMENTS

Obstacles, solutions, and thoughts on your progress.

_____

_____

_____

_____

I Did It!

DAILY GOALS
ACHIEVED

DATE:

WEIGHT:

WATER INTAKE:
# of 8oz. glasses

☐ ☐ ☐ ☐
☐ ☐ ☐ ☐

ENERGY LEVEL:

☐ low
☐ medium
☐ high

DAILY # OF SERVINGS:

fruits

veggies

grains

meats & beans

milk & dairy

oils & sweets

VITAMINS & SUPPLEMENTS:

DAILY NUTRITIONAL INTAKE

Food/Beverages	Qty.	Calories	Fat	Carbs.	Protein	Fiber
DAILY TOTALS:						

DAILY EXERCISE

Activity	Hrs./Mins.	Cal. Burned
DAILY TOTALS:		

TIP OF THE DAY!

Tracking your weight on a daily basis can help you keep a close eye on what eating patterns help you lose weight.

DAILY NOTES, ACHIEVEMENTS

Obstacles, solutions, and thoughts on your progress.

WEEKLY PROGRESS

12

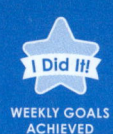

WEEKLY GOALS ACHIEVED

HIGHLIGHT OF THE WEEK

Your single-greatest moment of the week!

_____
_____
_____
_____

NUTRITIONAL INTAKE WRAP-UP

Did you meet your intake goals for the week? Why or why not?

_____
_____
_____
_____
_____
_____

EXERCISE WRAP-UP

Did you meet your exercise goals for the week? Why or why not?

_____
_____
_____
_____
_____

GOALS FOR NEXT WEEK

Things to work on for next week.

_____
_____
_____
_____
_____
_____
_____
_____

START WEIGHT:

END WEIGHT:

DAYS I TRACKED MY DIET:

- ☐ Mon.
- ☐ Tues.
- ☐ Wed.
- ☐ Thurs.
- ☐ Fri.
- ☐ Sat.
- ☐ Sun.

DAYS I EXERCISED:

- ☐ Mon.
- ☐ Tues.
- ☐ Wed.
- ☐ Thurs.
- ☐ Fri.
- ☐ Sat.
- ☐ Sun.

WEEKLY CALORIES BURNED:

WEEKLY ENERGY LEVEL:

- ☐ low
- ☐ medium
- ☐ high

I Did It!
DAILY GOALS ACHIEVED

WEEK
13

MONDAY

DATE:

WEIGHT:

WATER INTAKE:
# of 8oz. glasses
☐ ☐ ☐ ☐
☐ ☐ ☐ ☐

ENERGY LEVEL:
☐ low
☐ medium
☐ high

DAILY # OF SERVINGS:

fruits

veggies

grains

meats & beans

milk & dairy

oils & sweets

VITAMINS & SUPPLEMENTS:

DAILY NUTRITIONAL INTAKE						
Food/Beverages	Qty.	Calories	Fat	Carbs.	Protein	Fiber
DAILY TOTALS:						

DAILY EXERCISE		
Activity	Hrs./Mins.	Cal. Burned
DAILY TOTALS:		

TIP OF THE DAY!

Keep healthy snacks in your kitchen. That way, when you have the urge to munch on something, you will have better choices on hand.

DAILY NOTES, ACHIEVEMENTS

Obstacles, solutions, and thoughts on your progress.

TUESDAY

I Did It!

DAILY GOALS
ACHIEVED

DAILY NUTRITIONAL INTAKE

Food/Beverages	Qty.	Calories	Fat	Carbs.	Protein	Fiber
DAILY TOTALS:						

DATE:

WEIGHT:

WATER INTAKE:
# of 8oz. glasses
☐ ☐ ☐ ☐
☐ ☐ ☐ ☐

ENERGY LEVEL:
☐ low
☐ medium
☐ high

DAILY # OF SERVINGS:

fruits

veggies

grains

meats & beans

milk & dairy

oils & sweets

VITAMINS & SUPPLEMENTS:

DAILY EXERCISE

Activity	Hrs./Mins.	Cal. Burned
DAILY TOTALS:		

TIP OF THE DAY!

Fat is an important nutrient: Just make sure that the fat you consume is the healthy, unsaturated kind found in fish, nuts, and seeds.

DAILY NOTES, ACHIEVEMENTS

Obstacles, solutions, and thoughts on your progress.

I Did It!
DAILY GOALS
ACHIEVED

WEEK
13

WEDNESDAY

DATE:

WEIGHT:

WATER INTAKE:
# of 8oz. glasses

☐ ☐ ☐ ☐
☐ ☐ ☐ ☐

ENERGY LEVEL:

☐ low
☐ medium
☐ high

DAILY # OF SERVINGS:

fruits

veggies

grains

meats & beans

milk & dairy

oils & sweets

VITAMINS & SUPPLEMENTS:

DAILY NUTRITIONAL INTAKE

Food/Beverages	Qty.	Calories	Fat	Carbs.	Protein	Fiber
DAILY TOTALS:						

DAILY EXERCISE

Activity	Hrs./Mins.	Cal. Burned
DAILY TOTALS:		

TIP OF THE DAY!

Consider your resolution to lose weight as a benefit to yourself, not a test of your willpower.

DAILY NOTES, ACHIEVEMENTS

Obstacles, solutions, and thoughts on your progress.

THURSDAY

I Did It!

**DAILY GOALS
ACHIEVED**

DAILY NUTRITIONAL INTAKE

Food/Beverages	Qty.	Calories	Fat	Carbs.	Protein	Fiber
_____	____					
_____	____					
_____	____					
_____	____					
_____	____					
_____	____					
_____	____					
_____	____					
_____	____					
_____	____					
_____	____					
_____	____					
_____	____					
_____	____					
_____	____					
_____	____					
_____	____					
DAILY TOTALS:						

DATE:

WEIGHT:

WATER INTAKE:
# of 8oz. glasses

☐ ☐ ☐ ☐
☐ ☐ ☐ ☐

ENERGY LEVEL:

☐ low
☐ medium
☐ high

**DAILY # OF
SERVINGS:**

fruits

veggies

grains

meats &
beans

milk &
dairy

oils &
sweets

**VITAMINS &
SUPPLEMENTS:**

DAILY EXERCISE

Activity	Hrs./Mins.	Cal. Burned
_____	_____	
_____	_____	
_____	_____	
_____	_____	
DAILY TOTALS:		

TIP OF THE DAY!

If using butter or margarine in your meal, try to enjoy them in small portions and from a tub, rather than a stick.

DAILY NOTES, ACHIEVEMENTS

Obstacles, solutions, and thoughts on your progress.

_____

_____

_____

I Did It!
DAILY GOALS ACHIEVED

WEEK
13

FRIDAY

DATE:

WEIGHT:

WATER INTAKE:
# of 8oz. glasses
☐ ☐ ☐ ☐
☐ ☐ ☐ ☐

ENERGY LEVEL:
☐ low
☐ medium
☐ high

DAILY # OF SERVINGS:

fruits

veggies

grains

meats & beans

milk & dairy

oils & sweets

VITAMINS & SUPPLEMENTS:

DAILY NUTRITIONAL INTAKE

Food/Beverages	Qty.	Calories	Fat	Carbs.	Protein	Fiber
DAILY TOTALS:						

DAILY EXERCISE

Activity	Hrs./Mins.	Cal. Burned
DAILY TOTALS:		

TIP OF THE DAY!

Share your intentions to eat healthy with the people around you to create a sense of accountability.

DAILY NOTES, ACHIEVEMENTS

Obstacles, solutions, and thoughts on your progress.

SATURDAY

I Did It!

DAILY GOALS ACHIEVED

DAILY NUTRITIONAL INTAKE

Food/Beverages	Qty.	Calories	Fat	Carbs.	Protein	Fiber
_____	_____					
_____	_____					
_____	_____					
_____	_____					
_____	_____					
_____	_____					
_____	_____					
_____	_____					
_____	_____					
_____	_____					
_____	_____					
_____	_____					
_____	_____					
_____	_____					
_____	_____					
_____	_____					
DAILY TOTALS:						

DATE:

WEIGHT:

WATER INTAKE:
# of 8oz. glasses
☐ ☐ ☐ ☐
☐ ☐ ☐ ☐

ENERGY LEVEL:
☐ low
☐ medium
☐ high

DAILY # OF SERVINGS:

fruits

veggies

grains

meats & beans

milk & dairy

oils & sweets

DAILY EXERCISE

Activity	Hrs./Mins.	Cal. Burned
_____	_____	
_____	_____	
_____	_____	
_____	_____	
_____	_____	
DAILY TOTALS:		

TIP OF THE DAY!

If you are headed to a party where hors d'oeuvres and bowls of snacks will be served, try to eat a small meal beforehand.

VITAMINS & SUPPLEMENTS:

_____

_____

_____

_____

_____

DAILY NOTES, ACHIEVEMENTS

Obstacles, solutions, and thoughts on your progress.

_____

_____

_____

_____

I Did It!

DAILY GOALS
ACHIEVED

WEEK
13

SUNDAY

DATE:

WEIGHT:

WATER INTAKE:
# of 8oz. glasses

☐ ☐ ☐ ☐
☐ ☐ ☐ ☐

ENERGY LEVEL:

☐ low
☐ medium
☐ high

DAILY # OF SERVINGS:

fruits

veggies

grains

meats & beans

milk & dairy

oils & sweets

VITAMINS & SUPPLEMENTS:

DAILY NUTRITIONAL INTAKE						
Food/Beverages	Qty.	Calories	Fat	Carbs.	Protein	Fiber
DAILY TOTALS:						

DAILY EXERCISE		
Activity	Hrs./Mins.	Cal. Burned
DAILY TOTALS:		

TIP OF THE DAY!

Look for local or online weight-loss support communities where you can share your story, get tips, and ask for advice.

DAILY NOTES, ACHIEVEMENTS

Obstacles, solutions, and thoughts on your progress.

WEEKLY PROGRESS

WEEK
13

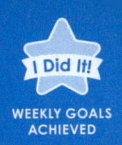

I Did It!

WEEKLY GOALS
ACHIEVED

HIGHLIGHT OF THE WEEK

Your single-greatest moment of the week!

_____

_____

_____

_____

START WEIGHT:

END WEIGHT:

NUTRITIONAL INTAKE WRAP-UP

Did you meet your intake goals for the week? Why or why not?

_____

_____

_____

_____

_____

_____

DAYS I TRACKED MY DIET:

☐ Mon.

☐ Tues.

☐ Wed.

☐ Thurs.

☐ Fri.

☐ Sat.

☐ Sun.

EXERCISE WRAP-UP

Did you meet your exercise goals for the week? Why or why not?

_____

_____

_____

_____

DAYS I EXERCISED:

☐ Mon.

☐ Tues.

☐ Wed.

☐ Thurs.

☐ Fri.

☐ Sat.

☐ Sun.

GOALS FOR NEXT WEEK

Things to work on for next week.

_____

_____

_____

_____

_____

_____

_____

_____

WEEKLY CALORIES BURNED:

WEEKLY ENERGY LEVEL:

☐ low

☐ medium

☐ high

I Did It!

DAILY GOALS
ACHIEVED

DATE:

WEIGHT:

WATER INTAKE:
# of 8oz. glasses

☐ ☐ ☐ ☐
☐ ☐ ☐ ☐

ENERGY LEVEL:

☐ low
☐ medium
☐ high

DAILY # OF SERVINGS:

fruits

veggies

grains

meats & beans

milk & dairy

oils & sweets

VITAMINS & SUPPLEMENTS:

DAILY NUTRITIONAL INTAKE

Food/Beverages	Qty.	Calories	Fat	Carbs.	Protein	Fiber

DAILY TOTALS:

DAILY EXERCISE

Activity	Hrs./Mins.	Cal. Burned

DAILY TOTALS:

TIP OF THE DAY!

Cereal is an excellent source of fiber. Check out the label for cereals that have at least 5 grams of fiber per serving.

DAILY NOTES, ACHIEVEMENTS

Obstacles, solutions, and thoughts on your progress.

TUESDAY

WEEK
14

I Did It!

**DAILY GOALS
ACHIEVED**

DAILY NUTRITIONAL INTAKE

Food/Beverages	Qty.	Calories	Fat	Carbs.	Protein	Fiber
_____	__					
_____	__					
_____	__					
_____	__					
_____	__					
_____	__					
_____	__					
_____	__					
_____	__					
_____	__					
_____	__					
_____	__					
_____	__					
_____	__					
_____	__					
_____	__					
_____	__					
_____	__					
DAILY TOTALS:						

DATE:

WEIGHT:

WATER INTAKE:
# of 8oz. glasses

☐ ☐ ☐ ☐
☐ ☐ ☐ ☐

ENERGY LEVEL:

☐ low
☐ medium
☐ high

**DAILY # OF
SERVINGS:**

fruits

veggies

grains

meats &
beans

milk &
dairy

oils &
sweets

**VITAMINS &
SUPPLEMENTS:**

DAILY EXERCISE

Activity	Hrs./Mins.	Cal. Burned
_____	___	
_____	___	
_____	___	
_____	___	
DAILY TOTALS:		

TIP OF THE DAY!

Enjoy an occasional
splurge, but mentally
prepare to go back
to your routine the
following day.

DAILY NOTES, ACHIEVEMENTS

Obstacles, solutions, and thoughts on your progress.

_____

_____

_____

I Did It!

DAILY GOALS
ACHIEVED

WEEK **14** **WEDNESDAY**

DATE:

WEIGHT:

WATER INTAKE:
# of 8oz. glasses

☐ ☐ ☐ ☐
☐ ☐ ☐ ☐

ENERGY LEVEL:

☐ low
☐ medium
☐ high

DAILY # OF SERVINGS:

fruits

veggies

grains

meats & beans

milk & dairy

oils & sweets

VITAMINS & SUPPLEMENTS:

DAILY NUTRITIONAL INTAKE

Food/Beverages	Qty.	Calories	Fat	Carbs.	Protein	Fiber
DAILY TOTALS:						

DAILY EXERCISE

Activity	Hrs./Mins.	Cal. Burned
DAILY TOTALS:		

TIP OF THE DAY!

Schedule rewards into your program to congratulate yourself for every positive step you make.

DAILY NOTES, ACHIEVEMENTS

Obstacles, solutions, and thoughts on your progress.

THURSDAY

I Did It!

DAILY GOALS
ACHIEVED

DAILY NUTRITIONAL INTAKE

Food/Beverages	Qty.	Calories	Fat	Carbs.	Protein	Fiber
DAILY TOTALS:						

DATE:

WEIGHT:

WATER INTAKE:
# of 8oz. glasses

ENERGY LEVEL:
- [ ] low
- [ ] medium
- [ ] high

DAILY # OF SERVINGS:
- fruits
- veggies
- grains
- meats & beans
- milk & dairy
- oils & sweets

VITAMINS & SUPPLEMENTS:

DAILY EXERCISE

Activity	Hrs./Mins.	Cal. Burned
DAILY TOTALS:		

TIP OF THE DAY!

Do not confuse water loss with fat loss.

DAILY NOTES, ACHIEVEMENTS

Obstacles, solutions, and thoughts on your progress.

I Did It!

DAILY GOALS ACHIEVED

WEEK
14

FRIDAY

DATE:

WEIGHT:

WATER INTAKE:
# of 8oz. glasses

☐ ☐ ☐ ☐
☐ ☐ ☐ ☐

ENERGY LEVEL:
☐ low
☐ medium
☐ high

DAILY # OF SERVINGS:

fruits

veggies

grains

meats & beans

milk & dairy

oils & sweets

VITAMINS & SUPPLEMENTS:

DAILY NUTRITIONAL INTAKE

Food/Beverages	Qty.	Calories	Fat	Carbs.	Protein	Fiber
DAILY TOTALS:						

DAILY EXERCISE

Activity	Hrs./Mins.	Cal. Burned
DAILY TOTALS:		

TIP OF THE DAY!

Eating a salad before the start of your meal can help curb your appetite, allowing you to eat smaller portions of your main course.

DAILY NOTES, ACHIEVEMENTS

Obstacles, solutions, and thoughts on your progress.

SATURDAY

I Did It!

DAILY GOALS
ACHIEVED

DAILY NUTRITIONAL INTAKE

Food/Beverages	Qty.	Calories	Fat	Carbs.	Protein	Fiber
DAILY TOTALS:						

DAILY EXERCISE

Activity	Hrs./Mins.	Cal. Burned
DAILY TOTALS:		

TIP OF THE DAY!

Start a moderate exercise routine by adding 10 to 15 minutes of aerobic activity to your daily schedule.

DAILY NOTES, ACHIEVEMENTS

Obstacles, solutions, and thoughts on your progress.

DATE:

WEIGHT:

WATER INTAKE:
# of 8oz. glasses

ENERGY LEVEL:
☐ low
☐ medium
☐ high

DAILY # OF SERVINGS:

fruits

veggies

grains

meats & beans

milk & dairy

oils & sweets

VITAMINS & SUPPLEMENTS:

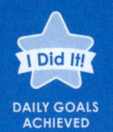

I Did It!
DAILY GOALS
ACHIEVED

WEEK
14

SUNDAY

DATE:

WEIGHT:

WATER INTAKE:
# of 8oz. glasses

☐ ☐ ☐ ☐
☐ ☐ ☐ ☐

ENERGY LEVEL:

☐ low
☐ medium
☐ high

DAILY # OF SERVINGS:

fruits

veggies

grains

meats & beans

milk & dairy

oils & sweets

VITAMINS & SUPPLEMENTS:

DAILY NUTRITIONAL INTAKE

Food/Beverages	Qty.	Calories	Fat	Carbs.	Protein	Fiber
DAILY TOTALS:						

DAILY EXERCISE

Activity	Hrs./Mins.	Cal. Burned
DAILY TOTALS:		

TIP OF THE DAY!

Realize that the last 5 pounds can be the most challenging to lose.

DAILY NOTES, ACHIEVEMENTS

Obstacles, solutions, and thoughts on your progress.

WEEKLY PROGRESS

WEEK
14

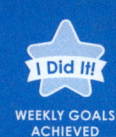

I Did It!

WEEKLY GOALS ACHIEVED

HIGHLIGHT OF THE WEEK

Your single-greatest moment of the week!

_____
_____
_____
_____
_____

NUTRITIONAL INTAKE WRAP-UP

Did you meet your intake goals for the week? Why or why not?

_____
_____
_____
_____
_____
_____
_____

EXERCISE WRAP-UP

Did you meet your exercise goals for the week? Why or why not?

_____
_____
_____
_____
_____

GOALS FOR NEXT WEEK

Things to work on for next week.

_____
_____
_____
_____
_____
_____
_____
_____
_____

START WEIGHT:

END WEIGHT:

DAYS I TRACKED MY DIET:

- [ ] Mon.
- [ ] Tues.
- [ ] Wed.
- [ ] Thurs.
- [ ] Fri.
- [ ] Sat.
- [ ] Sun.

DAYS I EXERCISED:

- [ ] Mon.
- [ ] Tues.
- [ ] Wed.
- [ ] Thurs.
- [ ] Fri.
- [ ] Sat.
- [ ] Sun.

WEEKLY CALORIES BURNED:

WEEKLY ENERGY LEVEL:

- [ ] low
- [ ] medium
- [ ] high

I Did It!
DAILY GOALS
ACHIEVED

MONDAY

DATE:

WEIGHT:

WATER INTAKE:
# of 8oz. glasses
☐ ☐ ☐ ☐
☐ ☐ ☐ ☐

ENERGY LEVEL:
☐ low
☐ medium
☐ high

DAILY # OF SERVINGS:

fruits

veggies

grains

meats & beans

milk & dairy

oils & sweets

VITAMINS & SUPPLEMENTS:

DAILY NUTRITIONAL INTAKE						
Food/Beverages	Qty.	Calories	Fat	Carbs.	Protein	Fiber
DAILY TOTALS:						

DAILY EXERCISE		
Activity	Hrs./Mins.	Cal. Burned
DAILY TOTALS:		

TIP OF THE DAY!

Instead of thinking of dieting as "giving up" foods, think of it as eating your favorite foods, but in moderation.

DAILY NOTES, ACHIEVEMENTS

Obstacles, solutions, and thoughts on your progress.

TUESDAY

I Did It!

DAILY GOALS
ACHIEVED

DAILY NUTRITIONAL INTAKE

Food/Beverages	Qty.	Calories	Fat	Carbs.	Protein	Fiber
DAILY TOTALS:						

DAILY EXERCISE

Activity	Hrs./Mins.	Cal. Burned
DAILY TOTALS:		

TIP OF THE DAY!

Smaller portion sizes and higher-calorie foods eaten in small amounts can help you lose weight without making you feel like you are depriving yourself.

DAILY NOTES, ACHIEVEMENTS

Obstacles, solutions, and thoughts on your progress.

_____

_____

_____

DATE:

WEIGHT:

WATER INTAKE:
# of 8oz. glasses
☐ ☐ ☐ ☐
☐ ☐ ☐ ☐

ENERGY LEVEL:
☐ low
☐ medium
☐ high

DAILY # OF SERVINGS:

fruits

veggies

grains

meats & beans

milk & dairy

oils & sweets

VITAMINS & SUPPLEMENTS:

_____

_____

_____

_____

_____

_____

I Did It!

DAILY GOALS ACHIEVED

WEEK
15

WEDNESDAY

DATE:

WEIGHT:

WATER INTAKE:
# of 8oz. glasses

☐ ☐ ☐ ☐
☐ ☐ ☐ ☐

ENERGY LEVEL:

☐ low
☐ medium
☐ high

DAILY # OF SERVINGS:

fruits

veggies

grains

meats & beans

milk & dairy

oils & sweets

VITAMINS & SUPPLEMENTS:

DAILY NUTRITIONAL INTAKE

Food/Beverages	Qty.	Calories	Fat	Carbs.	Protein	Fiber
DAILY TOTALS:						

DAILY EXERCISE

Activity	Hrs./Mins.	Cal. Burned
DAILY TOTALS:		

TIP OF THE DAY!

Make slow, small changes to your diet instead of fast, big changes. This way, your healthy lifestyle is easier to maintain.

DAILY NOTES, ACHIEVEMENTS

Obstacles, solutions, and thoughts on your progress.

THURSDAY

I Did It!

DAILY GOALS ACHIEVED

DAILY NUTRITIONAL INTAKE

Food/Beverages	Qty.	Calories	Fat	Carbs.	Protein	Fiber
DAILY TOTALS:						

DATE:

WEIGHT:

WATER INTAKE:
# of 8oz. glasses
☐ ☐ ☐ ☐
☐ ☐ ☐ ☐

ENERGY LEVEL:
☐ low
☐ medium
☐ high

DAILY # OF SERVINGS:
- fruits
- veggies
- grains
- meats & beans
- milk & dairy
- oils & sweets

VITAMINS & SUPPLEMENTS:

DAILY EXERCISE

Activity	Hrs./Mins.	Cal. Burned
DAILY TOTALS:		

TIP OF THE DAY!

Plan your meals ahead of time. That way, you won't be caught off-guard or forced to make unhealthy food choices.

DAILY NOTES, ACHIEVEMENTS

Obstacles, solutions, and thoughts on your progress.

I Did It!

DAILY GOALS ACHIEVED

WEEK
15

FRIDAY

DATE:

WEIGHT:

WATER INTAKE:
# of 8oz. glasses

☐ ☐ ☐ ☐
☐ ☐ ☐ ☐

ENERGY LEVEL:
☐ low
☐ medium
☐ high

DAILY # OF SERVINGS:

fruits

veggies

grains

meats & beans

milk & dairy

oils & sweets

VITAMINS & SUPPLEMENTS:

DAILY NUTRITIONAL INTAKE						
Food/Beverages	Qty.	Calories	Fat	Carbs.	Protein	Fiber
DAILY TOTALS:						

DAILY EXERCISE		
Activity	Hrs./Mins.	Cal. Burned
DAILY TOTALS:		

TIP OF THE DAY!

Skipping breakfast will actually train your body to store more fat when it senses you are not getting enough food.

DAILY NOTES, ACHIEVEMENTS

Obstacles, solutions, and thoughts on your progress.

SATURDAY

I Did It!

DAILY GOALS
ACHIEVED

DAILY NUTRITIONAL INTAKE

Food/Beverages	Qty.	Calories	Fat	Carbs.	Protein	Fiber
DAILY TOTALS:						

DAILY EXERCISE

Activity	Hrs./Mins.	Cal. Burned
DAILY TOTALS:		

TIP OF THE DAY!

Drinking 5 cups of green tea may burn 70 to 80 extra calories a day.

DAILY NOTES, ACHIEVEMENTS

Obstacles, solutions, and thoughts on your progress.

DATE:

WEIGHT:

WATER INTAKE:
# of 8oz. glasses

☐ ☐ ☐ ☐
☐ ☐ ☐ ☐

ENERGY LEVEL:

☐ low

☐ medium

☐ high

DAILY # OF SERVINGS:

fruits

veggies

grains

meats & beans

milk & dairy

oils & sweets

VITAMINS & SUPPLEMENTS:

I Did It!
DAILY GOALS
ACHIEVED

WEEK
15

SUNDAY

DATE:

WEIGHT:

WATER INTAKE:
# of 8oz. glasses

☐ ☐ ☐ ☐
☐ ☐ ☐ ☐

ENERGY LEVEL:
☐ low
☐ medium
☐ high

DAILY # OF SERVINGS:

fruits

veggies

grains

meats & beans

milk & dairy

oils & sweets

VITAMINS & SUPPLEMENTS:

DAILY NUTRITIONAL INTAKE

Food/Beverages	Qty.	Calories	Fat	Carbs.	Protein	Fiber
DAILY TOTALS:						

DAILY EXERCISE

Activity	Hrs./Mins.	Cal. Burned
DAILY TOTALS:		

TIP OF THE DAY!

Working out on an empty stomach, such as in the morning or before you eat dinner, will help you burn the maximum amount of fat and calories.

DAILY NOTES, ACHIEVEMENTS

Obstacles, solutions, and thoughts on your progress.

WEEKLY PROGRESS

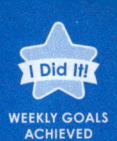

I Did It!

WEEKLY GOALS ACHIEVED

HIGHLIGHT OF THE WEEK

Your single-greatest moment of the week!

_____

_____

_____

_____

START WEIGHT:

END WEIGHT:

NUTRITIONAL INTAKE WRAP-UP

Did you meet your intake goals for the week? Why or why not?

_____

_____

_____

_____

_____

_____

_____

DAYS I TRACKED MY DIET:

- ☐ Mon.
- ☐ Tues.
- ☐ Wed.
- ☐ Thurs.
- ☐ Fri.
- ☐ Sat.
- ☐ Sun.

EXERCISE WRAP-UP

Did you meet your exercise goals for the week? Why or why not?

_____

_____

_____

_____

DAYS I EXERCISED:

- ☐ Mon.
- ☐ Tues.
- ☐ Wed.
- ☐ Thurs.
- ☐ Fri.
- ☐ Sat.
- ☐ Sun.

GOALS FOR NEXT WEEK

Things to work on for next week.

_____

_____

_____

_____

_____

_____

_____

_____

WEEKLY CALORIES BURNED:

WEEKLY ENERGY LEVEL:

- ☐ low
- ☐ medium
- ☐ high

MONTH
3

MONTHLY

DATE:

START WEIGHT:

END WEIGHT:

BODY FAT %:

MEASUREMENTS:

chest

biceps

waist

hips

thighs

NOTES:

PHOTO OF THE MONTH

Photo comments.

tape your photo here

PROGRESS

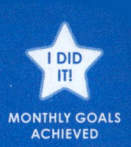

HIGHLIGHT OF THE MONTH

Your single-greatest moment of the month!

_____

_____

_____

_____

NUTRITIONAL INTAKE WRAP-UP

Did you meet your intake goals for the month? Why or why not?

_____

_____

_____

_____

_____

_____

EXERCISE WRAP-UP

Did you meet your exercise goals for the month? Why or why not?

_____

_____

_____

_____

_____

GOALS FOR NEXT MONTH

Things to work on for next month.

_____

_____

_____

_____

_____

_____

WEEK
16

MONDAY

DATE:

WEIGHT:

WATER INTAKE:
# of 8oz. glasses

☐ ☐ ☐ ☐
☐ ☐ ☐ ☐

ENERGY LEVEL:

☐ low
☐ medium
☐ high

**DAILY # OF
SERVINGS:**

fruits

veggies

grains

meats &
beans

milk &
dairy

oils &
sweets

**VITAMINS &
SUPPLEMENTS:**

DAILY NUTRITIONAL INTAKE

Food/Beverages	Qty.	Calories	Fat	Carbs.	Protein	Fiber
DAILY TOTALS:						

DAILY EXERCISE

Activity	Hrs./Mins.	Cal. Burned
DAILY TOTALS:		

TIP OF THE DAY!

If you need a burst of energy during your workout, have a snack with complex carbohydrates and protein handy, like a small piece of fruit and cheese.

DAILY NOTES, ACHIEVEMENTS

Obstacles, solutions, and thoughts on your progress.

TUESDAY

DAILY GOALS
ACHIEVED

DAILY NUTRITIONAL INTAKE

Food/Beverages	Qty.	Calories	Fat	Carbs.	Protein	Fiber
DAILY TOTALS:						

DAILY EXERCISE

Activity	Hrs./Mins.	Cal. Burned
DAILY TOTALS:		

TIP OF THE DAY!

Strive for consistency with your weight-loss program, not perfection.

DAILY NOTES, ACHIEVEMENTS

Obstacles, solutions, and thoughts on your progress.

_____
_____
_____
_____

DATE:

WEIGHT:

WATER INTAKE:
# of 8oz. glasses

☐ ☐ ☐ ☐
☐ ☐ ☐ ☐

ENERGY LEVEL:

☐ low
☐ medium
☐ high

DAILY # OF SERVINGS:

fruits

veggies

grains

meats & beans

milk & dairy

oils & sweets

VITAMINS & SUPPLEMENTS:

_____
_____
_____
_____
_____
_____

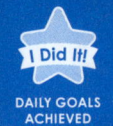
DATE:

WEIGHT:

WATER INTAKE:
# of 8oz. glasses

☐ ☐ ☐ ☐
☐ ☐ ☐ ☐

ENERGY LEVEL:
☐ low
☐ medium
☐ high

DAILY # OF SERVINGS:

fruits

veggies

grains

meats & beans

milk & dairy

oils & sweets

VITAMINS & SUPPLEMENTS:

DAILY NUTRITIONAL INTAKE

Food/Beverages	Qty.	Calories	Fat	Carbs.	Protein	Fiber
DAILY TOTALS:						

DAILY EXERCISE

Activity	Hrs./Mins.	Cal. Burned
DAILY TOTALS:		

TIP OF THE DAY!

Don't eat snack foods directly out of the package. Measure the portion you want to eat on a plate, and put the rest away.

DAILY NOTES, ACHIEVEMENTS

Obstacles, solutions, and thoughts on your progress.

THURSDAY

I Did It!

DAILY GOALS ACHIEVED

DAILY NUTRITIONAL INTAKE

Food/Beverages	Qty.	Calories	Fat	Carbs.	Protein	Fiber
_____	_____					
_____	_____					
_____	_____					
_____	_____					
_____	_____					
_____	_____					
_____	_____					
_____	_____					
_____	_____					
_____	_____					
_____	_____					
_____	_____					
_____	_____					
_____	_____					
_____	_____					
_____	_____					
_____	_____					
DAILY TOTALS:						

DATE:

WEIGHT:

WATER INTAKE:
# of 8oz. glasses

☐ ☐ ☐ ☐
☐ ☐ ☐ ☐

ENERGY LEVEL:

☐ low
☐ medium
☐ high

DAILY # OF SERVINGS:

fruits

veggies

grains

meats & beans

milk & dairy

oils & sweets

VITAMINS & SUPPLEMENTS:

DAILY EXERCISE

Activity	Hrs./Mins.	Cal. Burned
_____	_____	
_____	_____	
_____	_____	
_____	_____	
DAILY TOTALS:		

TIP OF THE DAY!

It takes 20 minutes for your brain to register that your stomach is full. If you eat slower while enjoying every bite, you are less likely to overeat.

DAILY NOTES, ACHIEVEMENTS

Obstacles, solutions, and thoughts on your progress.

_____
_____
_____

I Did It!
DAILY GOALS
ACHIEVED

FRIDAY

DATE:

WEIGHT:

WATER INTAKE:
# of 8oz. glasses

☐ ☐ ☐ ☐
☐ ☐ ☐ ☐

ENERGY LEVEL:
☐ low
☐ medium
☐ high

DAILY # OF SERVINGS:

fruits

veggies

grains

meats & beans

milk & dairy

oils & sweets

VITAMINS & SUPPLEMENTS:

DAILY NUTRITIONAL INTAKE

Food/Beverages	Qty.	Calories	Fat	Carbs.	Protein	Fiber
DAILY TOTALS:						

DAILY EXERCISE

Activity	Hrs./Mins.	Cal. Burned
DAILY TOTALS:		

TIP OF THE DAY!

Some research suggests that spicy foods, primarily red pepper, cayenne and chili pepper, may help raise your metabolism.

DAILY NOTES, ACHIEVEMENTS

Obstacles, solutions, and thoughts on your progress.

SATURDAY

I Did It!

DAILY GOALS
ACHIEVED

DAILY NUTRITIONAL INTAKE

Food/Beverages	Qty.	Calories	Fat	Carbs.	Protein	Fiber
DAILY TOTALS:						

DAILY EXERCISE

Activity	Hrs./Mins.	Cal. Burned
DAILY TOTALS:		

TIP OF THE DAY!

Plan ahead before going to the grocery store. Make a list of exactly what you want to buy, and don't spend time in the cookie or snack aisles.

DAILY NOTES, ACHIEVEMENTS

Obstacles, solutions, and thoughts on your progress.

DATE:

WEIGHT:

WATER INTAKE:
# of 8oz. glasses

☐ ☐ ☐ ☐
☐ ☐ ☐ ☐

ENERGY LEVEL:

☐ low
☐ medium
☐ high

DAILY # OF SERVINGS:

fruits

veggies

grains

meats & beans

milk & dairy

oils & sweets

VITAMINS & SUPPLEMENTS:

I Did It!

DAILY GOALS
ACHIEVED

DATE:

WEIGHT:

WATER INTAKE:
# of 8oz. glasses

☐ ☐ ☐ ☐
☐ ☐ ☐ ☐

ENERGY LEVEL:

☐ low
☐ medium
☐ high

DAILY # OF SERVINGS:

fruits

veggies

grains

meats & beans

milk & dairy

oils & sweets

VITAMINS & SUPPLEMENTS:

DAILY NUTRITIONAL INTAKE						
Food/Beverages	Qty.	Calories	Fat	Carbs.	Protein	Fiber
DAILY TOTALS:						

DAILY EXERCISE		
Activity	Hrs./Mins.	Cal. Burned
DAILY TOTALS:		

TIP OF THE DAY!

Create a healthy diet that focuses on unprocessed foods such as fruit, vegetables, whole grains, legumes, and lean protein.

DAILY NOTES, ACHIEVEMENTS

Obstacles, solutions, and thoughts on your progress.

WEEKLY PROGRESS WEEK 16

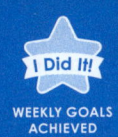

I Did It!
WEEKLY GOALS
ACHIEVED

HIGHLIGHT OF THE WEEK

Your single-greatest moment of the week!

_____
_____
_____
_____
_____

NUTRITIONAL INTAKE WRAP-UP

Did you meet your intake goals for the week? Why or why not?

_____
_____
_____
_____
_____
_____
_____

EXERCISE WRAP-UP

Did you meet your exercise goals for the week? Why or why not?

_____
_____
_____
_____
_____

GOALS FOR NEXT WEEK

Things to work on for next week.

_____
_____
_____
_____
_____
_____
_____

START WEIGHT:

END WEIGHT:

DAYS I TRACKED MY DIET:
- ☐ Mon.
- ☐ Tues.
- ☐ Wed.
- ☐ Thurs.
- ☐ Fri.
- ☐ Sat.
- ☐ Sun.

DAYS I EXERCISED:
- ☐ Mon.
- ☐ Tues.
- ☐ Wed.
- ☐ Thurs.
- ☐ Fri.
- ☐ Sat.
- ☐ Sun.

WEEKLY CALORIES BURNED:

WEEKLY ENERGY LEVEL:
- ☐ low
- ☐ medium
- ☐ high

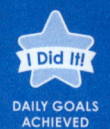

I Did It!
DAILY GOALS
ACHIEVED

MONDAY

DATE:

WEIGHT:

WATER INTAKE:
# of 8oz. glasses
☐ ☐ ☐ ☐
☐ ☐ ☐ ☐

ENERGY LEVEL:
☐ low
☐ medium
☐ high

DAILY # OF SERVINGS:

fruits

veggies

grains

meats & beans

milk & dairy

oils & sweets

VITAMINS & SUPPLEMENTS:

DAILY NUTRITIONAL INTAKE

Food/Beverages	Qty.	Calories	Fat	Carbs.	Protein	Fiber
DAILY TOTALS:						

DAILY EXERCISE

Activity	Hrs./Mins.	Cal. Burned
DAILY TOTALS:		

TIP OF THE DAY!

Tofu is a good substitute for many foods because it is rich in high-quality protein and contains no cholesterol. Try using it in place of cream in sauces.

DAILY NOTES, ACHIEVEMENTS

Obstacles, solutions, and thoughts on your progress.

TUESDAY

DAILY GOALS
ACHIEVED

DAILY NUTRITIONAL INTAKE

Food/Beverages	Qty.	Calories	Fat	Carbs.	Protein	Fiber
DAILY TOTALS:						

DAILY EXERCISE

Activity	Hrs./Mins.	Cal. Burned
DAILY TOTALS:		

TIP OF THE DAY!

Chicken broth and fresh herbs are an excellent and delicious substitute for butter and margarine when cooking.

DAILY NOTES, ACHIEVEMENTS

Obstacles, solutions, and thoughts on your progress.

_____
_____
_____

DATE:

WEIGHT:

WATER INTAKE:
# of 8oz. glasses
☐ ☐ ☐ ☐
☐ ☐ ☐ ☐

ENERGY LEVEL:
☐ low
☐ medium
☐ high

DAILY # OF SERVINGS:

fruits

veggies

grains

meats & beans

milk & dairy

oils & sweets

VITAMINS & SUPPLEMENTS:

_____
_____
_____
_____
_____
_____
_____

I Did It!
DAILY GOALS ACHIEVED

WEEK
17

WEDNESDAY

DATE:

WEIGHT:

WATER INTAKE:
# of 8oz. glasses

☐ ☐ ☐ ☐
☐ ☐ ☐ ☐

ENERGY LEVEL:
☐ low
☐ medium
☐ high

DAILY # OF SERVINGS:

fruits

veggies

grains

meats & beans

milk & dairy

oils & sweets

VITAMINS & SUPPLEMENTS:

DAILY NUTRITIONAL INTAKE

Food/Beverages	Qty.	Calories	Fat	Carbs.	Protein	Fiber
DAILY TOTALS:						

DAILY EXERCISE

Activity	Hrs./Mins.	Cal. Burned
DAILY TOTALS:		

TIP OF THE DAY!

Add lean protein to your diet, such as ground turkey, skinless white-meat poultry, as well as egg whites, fish, and legumes.

DAILY NOTES, ACHIEVEMENTS

Obstacles, solutions, and thoughts on your progress.

THURSDAY

DAILY GOALS ACHIEVED

DAILY NUTRITIONAL INTAKE

Food/Beverages	Qty.	Calories	Fat	Carbs.	Protein	Fiber
DAILY TOTALS:						

DAILY EXERCISE

Activity	Hrs./Mins.	Cal. Burned
DAILY TOTALS:		

TIP OF THE DAY!

After dinner or other large meals, try going for a long walk with a friend.

DAILY NOTES, ACHIEVEMENTS

Obstacles, solutions, and thoughts on your progress.

DATE:

WEIGHT:

WATER INTAKE:
# of 8oz. glasses

ENERGY LEVEL:
- [ ] low
- [ ] medium
- [ ] high

DAILY # OF SERVINGS:

- fruits
- veggies
- grains
- meats & beans
- milk & dairy
- oils & sweets

VITAMINS & SUPPLEMENTS:

I Did It!

DAILY GOALS
ACHIEVED

WEEK
17

FRIDAY

DATE:

WEIGHT:

WATER INTAKE:
# of 8oz. glasses

☐ ☐ ☐ ☐
☐ ☐ ☐ ☐

ENERGY LEVEL:

☐ low

☐ medium

☐ high

DAILY # OF SERVINGS:

fruits

veggies

grains

meats & beans

milk & dairy

oils & sweets

VITAMINS & SUPPLEMENTS:

DAILY NUTRITIONAL INTAKE						
Food/Beverages	Qty.	Calories	Fat	Carbs.	Protein	Fiber
DAILY TOTALS:						

DAILY EXERCISE		
Activity	Hrs./Mins.	Cal. Burned
DAILY TOTALS:		

TIP OF THE DAY!

Try to have something small to eat every 2 to 3 hours. Avoid large gaps of time without food where your hunger completely takes over.

DAILY NOTES, ACHIEVEMENTS

Obstacles, solutions, and thoughts on your progress.

SATURDAY

DAILY GOALS ACHIEVED

DAILY NUTRITIONAL INTAKE

Food/Beverages	Qty.	Calories	Fat	Carbs.	Protein	Fiber
DAILY TOTALS:						

DAILY EXERCISE

Activity	Hrs./Mins.	Cal. Burned
DAILY TOTALS:		

TIP OF THE DAY!

Each time you sit down to eat, think of it as a new opportunity to make healthy food choices!

DAILY NOTES, ACHIEVEMENTS

Obstacles, solutions, and thoughts on your progress.

DATE:

WEIGHT:

WATER INTAKE:
# of 8oz. glasses

☐ ☐ ☐ ☐
☐ ☐ ☐ ☐

ENERGY LEVEL:
☐ low
☐ medium
☐ high

DAILY # OF SERVINGS:
fruits
veggies
grains
meats & beans
milk & dairy
oils & sweets

VITAMINS & SUPPLEMENTS:

I Did It!

DAILY GOALS
ACHIEVED

WEEK 17

SUNDAY

DATE:

WEIGHT:

WATER INTAKE:
# of 8oz. glasses

☐ ☐ ☐ ☐
☐ ☐ ☐ ☐

ENERGY LEVEL:
☐ low
☐ medium
☐ high

DAILY # OF SERVINGS:

fruits

veggies

grains

meats & beans

milk & dairy

oils & sweets

VITAMINS & SUPPLEMENTS:

DAILY NUTRITIONAL INTAKE

Food/Beverages	Qty.	Calories	Fat	Carbs.	Protein	Fiber
DAILY TOTALS:						

DAILY EXERCISE

Activity	Hrs./Mins.	Cal. Burned
DAILY TOTALS:		

TIP OF THE DAY!

Burn more calories than you eat with nutrient- and fiber-dense foods like fruits and vegetables.

DAILY NOTES, ACHIEVEMENTS

Obstacles, solutions, and thoughts on your progress.

WEEKLY PROGRESS

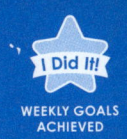

I Did It!
WEEKLY GOALS
ACHIEVED

HIGHLIGHT OF THE WEEK

Your single-greatest moment of the week!

_____

_____

_____

_____

NUTRITIONAL INTAKE WRAP-UP

Did you meet your intake goals for the week? Why or why not?

_____

_____

_____

_____

_____

_____

EXERCISE WRAP-UP

Did you meet your exercise goals for the week? Why or why not?

_____

_____

_____

_____

GOALS FOR NEXT WEEK

Things to work on for next week.

_____

_____

_____

_____

_____

_____

_____

START WEIGHT:

END WEIGHT:

DAYS I TRACKED MY DIET:
- [ ] Mon.
- [ ] Tues.
- [ ] Wed.
- [ ] Thurs.
- [ ] Fri.
- [ ] Sat.
- [ ] Sun.

DAYS I EXERCISED:
- [ ] Mon.
- [ ] Tues.
- [ ] Wed.
- [ ] Thurs.
- [ ] Fri.
- [ ] Sat.
- [ ] Sun.

WEEKLY CALORIES BURNED:

WEEKLY ENERGY LEVEL:
- [ ] low
- [ ] medium
- [ ] high

I Did It!
DAILY GOALS
ACHIEVED

WEEK 18

MONDAY

DATE:

WEIGHT:

WATER INTAKE:
# of 8oz. glasses

☐ ☐ ☐ ☐
☐ ☐ ☐ ☐

ENERGY LEVEL:
☐ low
☐ medium
☐ high

DAILY # OF SERVINGS:

fruits

veggies

grains

meats & beans

milk & dairy

oils & sweets

VITAMINS & SUPPLEMENTS:

_____
_____
_____
_____
_____

DAILY NUTRITIONAL INTAKE

Food/Beverages	Qty.	Calories	Fat	Carbs.	Protein	Fiber
DAILY TOTALS:						

DAILY EXERCISE

Activity	Hrs./Mins.	Cal. Burned
DAILY TOTALS:		

TIP OF THE DAY!

Choose snacks that are rich in vitamins and will give you the proper nutrients your body needs. That way, you won't just be consuming empty calories.

DAILY NOTES, ACHIEVEMENTS

Obstacles, solutions, and thoughts on your progress.

_____
_____
_____

TUESDAY

I Did It!

DAILY GOALS
ACHIEVED

DAILY NUTRITIONAL INTAKE

Food/Beverages	Qty.	Calories	Fat	Carbs.	Protein	Fiber
DAILY TOTALS:						

DAILY EXERCISE

Activity	Hrs./Mins.	Cal. Burned
DAILY TOTALS:		

DAILY NOTES, ACHIEVEMENTS

Obstacles, solutions, and thoughts on your progress.

TIP OF THE DAY!

Buy a healthy cookbook or food magazine. It will be filled with delicious recipes to help you cook healthier meals.

DATE:

WEIGHT:

WATER INTAKE:
# of 8oz. glasses

☐ ☐ ☐ ☐
☐ ☐ ☐ ☐

ENERGY LEVEL:
☐ low
☐ medium
☐ high

DAILY # OF SERVINGS:
fruits
veggies
grains
meats & beans
milk & dairy
oils & sweets

VITAMINS & SUPPLEMENTS:

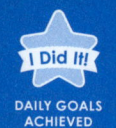

I Did It!

DAILY GOALS
ACHIEVED

WEEK 18 WEDNESDAY

DATE:

WEIGHT:

WATER INTAKE:
# of 8oz. glasses
☐ ☐ ☐ ☐
☐ ☐ ☐ ☐

ENERGY LEVEL:
☐ low
☐ medium
☐ high

DAILY # OF SERVINGS:

fruits

veggies

grains

meats & beans

milk & dairy

oils & sweets

VITAMINS & SUPPLEMENTS:

DAILY NUTRITIONAL INTAKE

Food/Beverages	Qty.	Calories	Fat	Carbs.	Protein	Fiber
DAILY TOTALS:						

DAILY EXERCISE

Activity	Hrs./Mins.	Cal. Burned
DAILY TOTALS:		

TIP OF THE DAY!

Eat soon after exercising to heal your body and restore energy.

DAILY NOTES, ACHIEVEMENTS

Obstacles, solutions, and thoughts on your progress.

THURSDAY

I Did It!

**DAILY GOALS
ACHIEVED**

DAILY NUTRITIONAL INTAKE

Food/Beverages	Qty.	Calories	Fat	Carbs.	Protein	Fiber
DAILY TOTALS:						

DATE:

WEIGHT:

WATER INTAKE:
# of 8oz. glasses
☐ ☐ ☐ ☐
☐ ☐ ☐ ☐

ENERGY LEVEL:
☐ low
☐ medium
☐ high

**DAILY # OF
SERVINGS:**

☐ fruits

☐ veggies

☐ grains

☐ meats &
beans

☐ milk &
dairy

☐ oils &
sweets

**VITAMINS &
SUPPLEMENTS:**

DAILY EXERCISE

Activity	Hrs./Mins.	Cal. Burned
DAILY TOTALS:		

TIP OF THE DAY!

When possible, take the stairs or park farther away from the store. Extra steps in your day mean extra calories burned over the long run.

DAILY NOTES, ACHIEVEMENTS

Obstacles, solutions, and thoughts on your progress.

I Did It!

DAILY GOALS
ACHIEVED

WEEK

18

FRIDAY

DATE:

WEIGHT:

WATER INTAKE:

# of 8oz. glasses

☐ ☐ ☐ ☐
☐ ☐ ☐ ☐

ENERGY LEVEL:

☐ low

☐ medium

☐ high

DAILY # OF SERVINGS:

fruits

veggies

grains

meats & beans

milk & dairy

oils & sweets

VITAMINS & SUPPLEMENTS:

DAILY NUTRITIONAL INTAKE

Food/Beverages	Qty.	Calories	Fat	Carbs.	Protein	Fiber
DAILY TOTALS:						

DAILY EXERCISE

Activity	Hrs./Mins.	Cal. Burned
DAILY TOTALS:		

TIP OF THE DAY!

Check-out aisles in grocery stores are laden with foods that are high in fat, calories, sugar, and salt; recognize this and resist temptation.

DAILY NOTES, ACHIEVEMENTS

Obstacles, solutions, and thoughts on your progress.

SATURDAY

I Did It!

DAILY GOALS ACHIEVED

DAILY NUTRITIONAL INTAKE

Food/Beverages	Qty.	Calories	Fat	Carbs.	Protein	Fiber
_____	____					
_____	____					
_____	____					
_____	____					
_____	____					
_____	____					
_____	____					
_____	____					
_____	____					
_____	____					
_____	____					
_____	____					
_____	____					
_____	____					
_____	____					
_____	____					
_____	____					
DAILY TOTALS:						

DATE:

WEIGHT:

WATER INTAKE:
# of 8oz. glasses

☐ ☐ ☐ ☐
☐ ☐ ☐ ☐

ENERGY LEVEL:
☐ low
☐ medium
☐ high

DAILY # OF SERVINGS:

fruits

veggies

grains

meats & beans

milk & dairy

oils & sweets

VITAMINS & SUPPLEMENTS:

DAILY EXERCISE

Activity	Hrs./Mins.	Cal. Burned
_____	____	
_____	____	
_____	____	
_____	____	
_____	____	
DAILY TOTALS:		

TIP OF THE DAY!

If joining a gym is not your thing, try organizing a game of basketball or Frisbee. Take a jog outdoors or walk your dog, if the weather is nice.

DAILY NOTES, ACHIEVEMENTS

Obstacles, solutions, and thoughts on your progress.

_____

_____

_____

I Did It!
DAILY GOALS
ACHIEVED

WEEK
18

SUNDAY

DATE:

WEIGHT:

WATER INTAKE:
# of 8oz. glasses
☐ ☐ ☐ ☐
☐ ☐ ☐ ☐

ENERGY LEVEL:
☐ low
☐ medium
☐ high

DAILY # OF SERVINGS:

fruits

veggies

grains

meats & beans

milk & dairy

oils & sweets

VITAMINS & SUPPLEMENTS:

DAILY NUTRITIONAL INTAKE

Food/Beverages	Qty.	Calories	Fat	Carbs.	Protein	Fiber
DAILY TOTALS:						

DAILY EXERCISE

Activity	Hrs./Mins.	Cal. Burned
DAILY TOTALS:		

TIP OF THE DAY!

Prepare your own meals as often as you can. You can control exactly what goes into each meal if you make it yourself.

DAILY NOTES, ACHIEVEMENTS

Obstacles, solutions, and thoughts on your progress.

WEEKLY PROGRESS

18

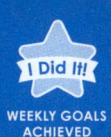

I Did It!

WEEKLY GOALS ACHIEVED

HIGHLIGHT OF THE WEEK

Your single-greatest moment of the week!

_____

_____

_____

_____

START WEIGHT:

END WEIGHT:

NUTRITIONAL INTAKE WRAP-UP

Did you meet your intake goals for the week? Why or why not?

_____

_____

_____

_____

_____

_____

DAYS I TRACKED MY DIET:

☐ Mon.

☐ Tues.

☐ Wed.

☐ Thurs.

☐ Fri.

☐ Sat.

☐ Sun.

EXERCISE WRAP-UP

Did you meet your exercise goals for the week? Why or why not?

_____

_____

_____

_____

_____

DAYS I EXERCISED:

☐ Mon.

☐ Tues.

☐ Wed.

☐ Thurs.

☐ Fri.

☐ Sat.

☐ Sun.

GOALS FOR NEXT WEEK

Things to work on for next week.

_____

_____

_____

_____

_____

_____

WEEKLY CALORIES BURNED:

WEEKLY ENERGY LEVEL:

☐ low

☐ medium

☐ high

I Did It!
DAILY GOALS ACHIEVED

DATE:

WEIGHT:

WATER INTAKE:
# of 8oz. glasses
☐ ☐ ☐ ☐
☐ ☐ ☐ ☐

ENERGY LEVEL:
☐ low
☐ medium
☐ high

DAILY # OF SERVINGS:

fruits

veggies

grains

meats & beans

milk & dairy

oils & sweets

VITAMINS & SUPPLEMENTS:

DAILY NUTRITIONAL INTAKE

Food/Beverages	Qty.	Calories	Fat	Carbs.	Protein	Fiber
DAILY TOTALS:						

DAILY EXERCISE

Activity	Hrs./Mins.	Cal. Burned
DAILY TOTALS:		

TIP OF THE DAY!

Don't think of how much more weight you have to lose, but rather think about how much you've already lost!

DAILY NOTES, ACHIEVEMENTS

Obstacles, solutions, and thoughts on your progress.

TUESDAY

I Did It!

DAILY GOALS
ACHIEVED

DAILY NUTRITIONAL INTAKE

Food/Beverages	Qty.	Calories	Fat	Carbs.	Protein	Fiber
_____	_____					
_____	_____					
_____	_____					
_____	_____					
_____	_____					
_____	_____					
_____	_____					
_____	_____					
_____	_____					
_____	_____					
_____	_____					
_____	_____					
_____	_____					
_____	_____					
_____	_____					
_____	_____					
_____	_____					
DAILY TOTALS:						

DATE:

WEIGHT:

WATER INTAKE:
# of 8oz. glasses
☐ ☐ ☐ ☐
☐ ☐ ☐ ☐

ENERGY LEVEL:
☐ low
☐ medium
☐ high

DAILY # OF
SERVINGS:

fruits

veggies

grains

meats &
beans

milk &
dairy

oils &
sweets

VITAMINS &
SUPPLEMENTS:

DAILY EXERCISE

Activity	Hrs./Mins.	Cal. Burned
_____	_____	
_____	_____	
_____	_____	
_____	_____	
_____	_____	
DAILY TOTALS:		

TIP OF THE DAY!

Congratulate yourself
every time you get a
step closer to your
weight-loss goal.

DAILY NOTES, ACHIEVEMENTS

Obstacles, solutions, and thoughts on your progress.

_____

_____

_____

I Did It!

DAILY GOALS
ACHIEVED

DATE:

WEIGHT:

WATER INTAKE:
# of 8oz. glasses

☐ ☐ ☐ ☐
☐ ☐ ☐ ☐

ENERGY LEVEL:

☐ low
☐ medium
☐ high

DAILY # OF SERVINGS:

fruits

veggies

grains

meats & beans

milk & dairy

oils & sweets

VITAMINS & SUPPLEMENTS:

DAILY NUTRITIONAL INTAKE

Food/Beverages	Qty.	Calories	Fat	Carbs.	Protein	Fiber
DAILY TOTALS:						

DAILY EXERCISE

Activity	Hrs./Mins.	Cal. Burned
DAILY TOTALS:		

TIP OF THE DAY!

Don't rule out foods because of the time of day. Make eggs for dinner or incorporate lean chicken in your omelet at breakfast.

DAILY NOTES, ACHIEVEMENTS

Obstacles, solutions, and thoughts on your progress.

THURSDAY

I Did It!

DAILY GOALS
ACHIEVED

DAILY NUTRITIONAL INTAKE

Food/Beverages	Qty.	Calories	Fat	Carbs.	Protein	Fiber
DAILY TOTALS:						

DATE:

WEIGHT:

WATER INTAKE:
# of 8oz. glasses

ENERGY LEVEL:
☐ low
☐ medium
☐ high

DAILY # OF
SERVINGS:
fruits
veggies
grains
meats &
beans
milk &
dairy
oils &
sweets

VITAMINS &
SUPPLEMENTS:

DAILY EXERCISE

Activity	Hrs./Mins.	Cal. Burned
DAILY TOTALS:		

TIP OF THE DAY!

Avoid going to a candy store or an ice cream shop where you will be tempted to stray from your diet.

DAILY NOTES, ACHIEVEMENTS

Obstacles, solutions, and thoughts on your progress.

I Did It!
DAILY GOALS ACHIEVED

WEEK
19

FRIDAY

DATE:

WEIGHT:

WATER INTAKE:
# of 8oz. glasses

☐ ☐ ☐ ☐
☐ ☐ ☐ ☐

ENERGY LEVEL:
☐ low
☐ medium
☐ high

DAILY # OF SERVINGS:

fruits

veggies

grains

meats & beans

milk & dairy

oils & sweets

VITAMINS & SUPPLEMENTS:

DAILY NUTRITIONAL INTAKE

Food/Beverages	Qty.	Calories	Fat	Carbs.	Protein	Fiber
DAILY TOTALS:						

DAILY EXERCISE

Activity	Hrs./Mins.	Cal. Burned
DAILY TOTALS:		

TIP OF THE DAY!

Instead of simply swearing off chips, cookies, cake, or candy, find healthy alternatives and have them available when you feel like snacking.

DAILY NOTES, ACHIEVEMENTS

Obstacles, solutions, and thoughts on your progress.

SATURDAY

I Did It!

DAILY GOALS
ACHIEVED

DAILY NUTRITIONAL INTAKE

Food/Beverages	Qty.	Calories	Fat	Carbs.	Protein	Fiber
DAILY TOTALS:						

DAILY EXERCISE

Activity	Hrs./Mins.	Cal. Burned
DAILY TOTALS:		

TIP OF THE DAY!

Walking at least 3 miles a day can contribute significantly to your weight-loss program.

DAILY NOTES, ACHIEVEMENTS

Obstacles, solutions, and thoughts on your progress.

DATE:

WEIGHT:

WATER INTAKE:
# of 8oz. glasses

☐ ☐ ☐ ☐
☐ ☐ ☐ ☐

ENERGY LEVEL:

☐ low

☐ medium

☐ high

DAILY # OF SERVINGS:

fruits

veggies

grains

meats & beans

milk & dairy

oils & sweets

VITAMINS & SUPPLEMENTS:

I Did It!

DAILY GOALS
ACHIEVED

SUNDAY

DATE:

WEIGHT:

WATER INTAKE:
# of 8oz. glasses

☐ ☐ ☐ ☐
☐ ☐ ☐ ☐

ENERGY LEVEL:

☐ low
☐ medium
☐ high

DAILY # OF SERVINGS:

fruits

veggies

grains

meats & beans

milk & dairy

oils & sweets

VITAMINS & SUPPLEMENTS:

DAILY NUTRITIONAL INTAKE

Food/Beverages	Qty.	Calories	Fat	Carbs.	Protein	Fiber
DAILY TOTALS:						

DAILY EXERCISE

Activity	Hrs./Mins.	Cal. Burned
DAILY TOTALS:		

TIP OF THE DAY!

Stock your freezer with healthy frozen entrees. Choose ones that are low in calories and low in sodium.

DAILY NOTES, ACHIEVEMENTS

Obstacles, solutions, and thoughts on your progress.

WEEKLY PROGRESS WEEK 19

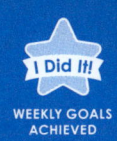

I Did It!

WEEKLY GOALS
ACHIEVED

HIGHLIGHT OF THE WEEK

Your single-greatest moment of the week!

_____

_____

_____

_____

_____

START WEIGHT:

END WEIGHT:

NUTRITIONAL INTAKE WRAP-UP

Did you meet your intake goals for the week? Why or why not?

_____

_____

_____

_____

_____

_____

_____

DAYS I TRACKED MY DIET:

☐ Mon.
☐ Tues.
☐ Wed.
☐ Thurs.
☐ Fri.
☐ Sat.
☐ Sun.

EXERCISE WRAP-UP

Did you meet your exercise goals for the week? Why or why not?

_____

_____

_____

_____

_____

DAYS I EXERCISED:

☐ Mon.
☐ Tues.
☐ Wed.
☐ Thurs.
☐ Fri.
☐ Sat.
☐ Sun.

GOALS FOR NEXT WEEK

Things to work on for next week.

_____

_____

_____

_____

_____

_____

_____

WEEKLY CALORIES BURNED:

WEEKLY ENERGY LEVEL:

☐ low
☐ medium
☐ high

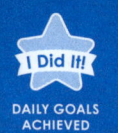

I Did It!
DAILY GOALS
ACHIEVED

MONDAY

DATE:

WEIGHT:

WATER INTAKE:
# of 8oz. glasses

☐ ☐ ☐ ☐
☐ ☐ ☐ ☐

ENERGY LEVEL:
☐ low
☐ medium
☐ high

DAILY # OF SERVINGS:

fruits

veggies

grains

meats & beans

milk & dairy

oils & sweets

VITAMINS & SUPPLEMENTS:

DAILY NUTRITIONAL INTAKE

Food/Beverages	Qty.	Calories	Fat	Carbs.	Protein	Fiber
DAILY TOTALS:						

DAILY EXERCISE

Activity	Hrs./Mins.	Cal. Burned
DAILY TOTALS:		

TIP OF THE DAY!

Add strength training to your aerobic workout. You will burn fat faster in the areas you build muscle.

DAILY NOTES, ACHIEVEMENTS

Obstacles, solutions, and thoughts on your progress.

TUESDAY

I Did It!

**DAILY GOALS
ACHIEVED**

DAILY NUTRITIONAL INTAKE

Food/Beverages	Qty.	Calories	Fat	Carbs.	Protein	Fiber
DAILY TOTALS:						

DAILY EXERCISE

Activity	Hrs./Mins.	Cal. Burned
DAILY TOTALS:		

TIP OF THE DAY!

Before strength training, consult a trainer who can guide you in the safety procedures and correct way to use exercise machines.

DAILY NOTES, ACHIEVEMENTS

Obstacles, solutions, and thoughts on your progress.

DATE:

WEIGHT:

WATER INTAKE:

# of 8oz. glasses

☐ ☐ ☐ ☐
☐ ☐ ☐ ☐

ENERGY LEVEL:

☐ low
☐ medium
☐ high

DAILY # OF SERVINGS:

fruits

veggies

grains

meats & beans

milk & dairy

oils & sweets

VITAMINS & SUPPLEMENTS:

I Did It!
DAILY GOALS
ACHIEVED

WEDNESDAY

DATE:

WEIGHT:

WATER INTAKE:
# of 8oz. glasses
☐ ☐ ☐ ☐
☐ ☐ ☐ ☐

ENERGY LEVEL:
☐ low
☐ medium
☐ high

DAILY # OF SERVINGS:

fruits

veggies

grains

meats & beans

milk & dairy

oils & sweets

VITAMINS & SUPPLEMENTS:

DAILY NUTRITIONAL INTAKE

Food/Beverages	Qty.	Calories	Fat	Carbs.	Protein	Fiber
DAILY TOTALS:						

DAILY EXERCISE

Activity	Hrs./Mins.	Cal. Burned
DAILY TOTALS:		

TIP OF THE DAY!

You won't need to rely on take-out, fast food, or delivery if your kitchen is stocked with nutritious foods that are easy to prepare.

DAILY NOTES, ACHIEVEMENTS

Obstacles, solutions, and thoughts on your progress.

THURSDAY

I Did It!

**DAILY GOALS
ACHIEVED**

DAILY NUTRITIONAL INTAKE

Food/Beverages	Qty.	Calories	Fat	Carbs.	Protein	Fiber
_____	____					
_____	____					
_____	____					
_____	____					
_____	____					
_____	____					
_____	____					
_____	____					
_____	____					
_____	____					
_____	____					
_____	____					
_____	____					
_____	____					
_____	____					
_____	____					
DAILY TOTALS:						

DATE:

WEIGHT:

WATER INTAKE:
# of 8oz. glasses
☐ ☐ ☐ ☐
☐ ☐ ☐ ☐

ENERGY LEVEL:
☐ low
☐ medium
☐ high

**DAILY # OF
SERVINGS:**
- fruits
- veggies
- grains
- meats &
  beans
- milk &
  dairy
- oils &
  sweets

**VITAMINS &
SUPPLEMENTS:**
_____
_____
_____
_____
_____
_____
_____

DAILY EXERCISE

Activity	Hrs./Mins.	Cal. Burned
_____	_____	
_____	_____	
_____	_____	
_____	_____	
_____	_____	
DAILY TOTALS:		

TIP OF THE DAY!

Don't cut too many
calories out of
your diet. If you
feel deprived or
unsatisfied, you are
more likely to cheat.

DAILY NOTES, ACHIEVEMENTS

Obstacles, solutions, and thoughts on your progress.

_____

_____

_____

I Did It!
DAILY GOALS
ACHIEVED

DATE:

WEIGHT:

WATER INTAKE:
# of 8oz. glasses

☐ ☐ ☐ ☐
☐ ☐ ☐ ☐

ENERGY LEVEL:
☐ low
☐ medium
☐ high

DAILY # OF SERVINGS:

fruits

veggies

grains

meats & beans

milk & dairy

oils & sweets

VITAMINS & SUPPLEMENTS:

DAILY NUTRITIONAL INTAKE

Food/Beverages	Qty.	Calories	Fat	Carbs.	Protein	Fiber
DAILY TOTALS:						

DAILY EXERCISE

Activity	Hrs./Mins.	Cal. Burned
DAILY TOTALS:		

TIP OF THE DAY!

Include a healthy treat into your weight-loss plan so you don't feel deprived. Try to keep these foods between 200 and 250 calories.

DAILY NOTES, ACHIEVEMENTS

Obstacles, solutions, and thoughts on your progress.

SATURDAY

I Did It!

DAILY GOALS ACHIEVED

DAILY NUTRITIONAL INTAKE

Food/Beverages	Qty.	Calories	Fat	Carbs.	Protein	Fiber
DAILY TOTALS:						

DATE:

WEIGHT:

WATER INTAKE:
# of 8oz. glasses

☐ ☐ ☐ ☐
☐ ☐ ☐ ☐

ENERGY LEVEL:

☐ low
☐ medium
☐ high

DAILY # OF SERVINGS:

fruits

veggies

grains

meats & beans

milk & dairy

oils & sweets

VITAMINS & SUPPLEMENTS:

DAILY EXERCISE

Activity	Hrs./Mins.	Cal. Burned
DAILY TOTALS:		

TIP OF THE DAY!

Varying your physical activity keeps your workout routine interesting and fun and keeps your body working at its peak potential.

DAILY NOTES, ACHIEVEMENTS

Obstacles, solutions, and thoughts on your progress.

I Did It!

DAILY GOALS ACHIEVED

WEEK
20

SUNDAY

DATE:

WEIGHT:

WATER INTAKE:
# of 8oz. glasses

☐ ☐ ☐ ☐
☐ ☐ ☐ ☐

ENERGY LEVEL:

☐ low
☐ medium
☐ high

DAILY # OF SERVINGS:

fruits

veggies

grains

meats & beans

milk & dairy

oils & sweets

VITAMINS & SUPPLEMENTS:

DAILY NUTRITIONAL INTAKE						
Food/Beverages	Qty.	Calories	Fat	Carbs.	Protein	Fiber
DAILY TOTALS:						

DAILY EXERCISE		
Activity	Hrs./Mins.	Cal. Burned
DAILY TOTALS:		

TIP OF THE DAY!

Make a list of all the foods you like that fit within your diet program so you can easily plan meals.

DAILY NOTES, ACHIEVEMENTS

Obstacles, solutions, and thoughts on your progress.

WEEKLY PROGRESS

WEEK 20

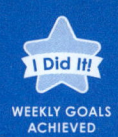

I Did It!

WEEKLY GOALS
ACHIEVED

HIGHLIGHT OF THE WEEK

Your single-greatest moment of the week!

_____
_____
_____
_____

NUTRITIONAL INTAKE WRAP-UP

Did you meet your intake goals for the week? Why or why not?

_____
_____
_____
_____
_____
_____

EXERCISE WRAP-UP

Did you meet your exercise goals for the week? Why or why not?

_____
_____
_____
_____
_____

GOALS FOR NEXT WEEK

Things to work on for next week.

_____
_____
_____
_____
_____
_____
_____

START WEIGHT:

END WEIGHT:

DAYS I TRACKED MY DIET:

☐ Mon.
☐ Tues.
☐ Wed.
☐ Thurs.
☐ Fri.
☐ Sat.
☐ Sun.

DAYS I EXERCISED:

☐ Mon.
☐ Tues.
☐ Wed.
☐ Thurs.
☐ Fri.
☐ Sat.
☐ Sun.

WEEKLY CALORIES BURNED:

WEEKLY ENERGY LEVEL:

☐ low
☐ medium
☐ high

MONTH 4

MONTHLY

DATE:

START WEIGHT:

END WEIGHT:

BODY FAT %:

MEASUREMENTS:

chest

biceps

waist

hips

thighs

NOTES:

PHOTO OF THE MONTH

Photo comments.

tape your photo here

PROGRESS

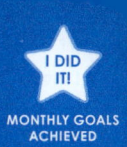

I DID IT!

MONTHLY GOALS ACHIEVED

HIGHLIGHT OF THE MONTH

Your single-greatest moment of the month!

_____
_____
_____
_____
_____

NUTRITIONAL INTAKE WRAP-UP

Did you meet your intake goals for the month? Why or why not?

_____
_____
_____
_____
_____
_____
_____

EXERCISE WRAP-UP

Did you meet your exercise goals for the month? Why or why not?

_____
_____
_____
_____
_____

GOALS FOR NEXT MONTH

Things to work on for next month.

_____
_____
_____
_____
_____
_____
_____

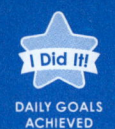

I Did It!
DAILY GOALS
ACHIEVED

DATE:

WEIGHT:

WATER INTAKE:
# of 8oz. glasses

☐ ☐ ☐ ☐
☐ ☐ ☐ ☐

ENERGY LEVEL:
☐ low
☐ medium
☐ high

DAILY # OF SERVINGS:

fruits

veggies

grains

meats & beans

milk & dairy

oils & sweets

VITAMINS & SUPPLEMENTS:

_____

_____

_____

_____

_____

_____

DAILY NUTRITIONAL INTAKE

Food/Beverages	Qty.	Calories	Fat	Carbs.	Protein	Fiber
DAILY TOTALS:						

DAILY EXERCISE

Activity	Hrs./Mins.	Cal. Burned
DAILY TOTALS:		

TIP OF THE DAY!

Look into joining fitness classes at your local gym. Working out with other people is a great way to stay motivated.

DAILY NOTES, ACHIEVEMENTS

Obstacles, solutions, and thoughts on your progress.

_____

_____

_____

TUESDAY

I Did It!
DAILY GOALS ACHIEVED

DAILY NUTRITIONAL INTAKE

Food/Beverages	Qty.	Calories	Fat	Carbs.	Protein	Fiber
DAILY TOTALS:						

DATE:

WEIGHT:

WATER INTAKE:
# of 8oz. glasses

☐ ☐ ☐ ☐
☐ ☐ ☐ ☐

ENERGY LEVEL:

☐ low
☐ medium
☐ high

DAILY # OF SERVINGS:

fruits

veggies

grains

meats & beans

milk & dairy

oils & sweets

VITAMINS & SUPPLEMENTS:

DAILY EXERCISE

Activity	Hrs./Mins.	Cal. Burned
DAILY TOTALS:		

TIP OF THE DAY!

After exercising, try stretching or another low-intensity activity for 10 minutes to gradually return your body to its pre-exercise state.

DAILY NOTES, ACHIEVEMENTS

Obstacles, solutions, and thoughts on your progress.

I Did It!

DAILY GOALS
ACHIEVED

DATE:

WEIGHT:

WATER INTAKE:
# of 8oz. glasses

☐ ☐ ☐ ☐
☐ ☐ ☐ ☐

ENERGY LEVEL:

☐ low
☐ medium
☐ high

DAILY # OF SERVINGS:

fruits

veggies

grains

meats & beans

milk & dairy

oils & sweets

VITAMINS & SUPPLEMENTS:

DAILY NUTRITIONAL INTAKE

Food/Beverages	Qty.	Calories	Fat	Carbs.	Protein	Fiber
DAILY TOTALS:						

DAILY EXERCISE

Activity	Hrs./Mins.	Cal. Burned
DAILY TOTALS:		

TIP OF THE DAY!

Have portable, healthy snacks on hand when you are stuck at the airport or are faced with a long flight.

DAILY NOTES, ACHIEVEMENTS

Obstacles, solutions, and thoughts on your progress.

THURSDAY

I Did It!

DAILY GOALS
ACHIEVED

DAILY NUTRITIONAL INTAKE

Food/Beverages	Qty.	Calories	Fat	Carbs.	Protein	Fiber
_____	___					
_____	___					
_____	___					
_____	___					
_____	___					
_____	___					
_____	___					
_____	___					
_____	___					
_____	___					
_____	___					
_____	___					
_____	___					
_____	___					
_____	___					
DAILY TOTALS:						

DATE:

WEIGHT:

WATER INTAKE:
# of 8oz. glasses

☐ ☐ ☐ ☐
☐ ☐ ☐ ☐

ENERGY LEVEL:

☐ low

☐ medium

☐ high

DAILY # OF SERVINGS:

fruits

veggies

grains

meats & beans

milk & dairy

oils & sweets

VITAMINS & SUPPLEMENTS:

_____
_____
_____
_____
_____
_____
_____

DAILY EXERCISE

Activity	Hrs./Mins.	Cal. Burned
_____	___	
_____	___	
_____	___	
_____	___	
_____	___	
DAILY TOTALS:		

TIP OF THE DAY!

If you're traveling, use the stairs and walk as much as possible. Or, try to book a hotel room with a fitness facility.

DAILY NOTES, ACHIEVEMENTS

Obstacles, solutions, and thoughts on your progress.

_____

_____

_____

I Did It!

DAILY GOALS ACHIEVED

WEEK 21

FRIDAY

DATE:

WEIGHT:

WATER INTAKE:
# of 8oz. glasses

☐ ☐ ☐ ☐
☐ ☐ ☐ ☐

ENERGY LEVEL:

☐ low

☐ medium

☐ high

DAILY # OF SERVINGS:

fruits

veggies

grains

meats & beans

milk & dairy

oils & sweets

VITAMINS & SUPPLEMENTS:

DAILY NUTRITIONAL INTAKE						
Food/Beverages	Qty.	Calories	Fat	Carbs.	Protein	Fiber
DAILY TOTALS:						

DAILY EXERCISE		
Activity	Hrs./Mins.	Cal. Burned
DAILY TOTALS:		

TIP OF THE DAY!

Losing weight while traveling is possible if you create an itinerary where you have healthy dining options at all stages of your trip.

DAILY NOTES, ACHIEVEMENTS

Obstacles, solutions, and thoughts on your progress.

SATURDAY

I Did It!

**DAILY GOALS
ACHIEVED**

DAILY NUTRITIONAL INTAKE

Food/Beverages	Qty.	Calories	Fat	Carbs.	Protein	Fiber
DAILY TOTALS:						

DAILY EXERCISE

Activity	Hrs./Mins.	Cal. Burned
DAILY TOTALS:		

TIP OF THE DAY!

Increase the intensity of your workouts only when your body is ready. Trying to force too much, too soon can potentially harm your body.

DAILY NOTES, ACHIEVEMENTS

Obstacles, solutions, and thoughts on your progress.

DATE:

WEIGHT:

WATER INTAKE:
# of 8oz. glasses
☐ ☐ ☐ ☐
☐ ☐ ☐ ☐

ENERGY LEVEL:
☐ low
☐ medium
☐ high

DAILY # OF SERVINGS:

fruits

veggies

grains

meats & beans

milk & dairy

oils & sweets

VITAMINS & SUPPLEMENTS:

I Did It!
DAILY GOALS
ACHIEVED

DATE:

WEIGHT:

WATER INTAKE:
# of 8oz. glasses

☐ ☐ ☐ ☐
☐ ☐ ☐ ☐

ENERGY LEVEL:
☐ low
☐ medium
☐ high

DAILY # OF SERVINGS:

fruits

veggies

grains

meats & beans

milk & dairy

oils & sweets

VITAMINS & SUPPLEMENTS:

DAILY NUTRITIONAL INTAKE

Food/Beverages	Qty.	Calories	Fat	Carbs.	Protein	Fiber
DAILY TOTALS:						

DAILY EXERCISE

Activity	Hrs./Mins.	Cal. Burned
DAILY TOTALS:		

TIP OF THE DAY!

Keep some meal replacement options in your car and at work.

DAILY NOTES, ACHIEVEMENTS

Obstacles, solutions, and thoughts on your progress.

WEEKLY PROGRESS
WEEK
21

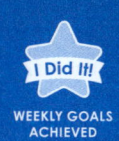
I Did It!
WEEKLY GOALS ACHIEVED

HIGHLIGHT OF THE WEEK

Your single-greatest moment of the week!

_____
_____
_____
_____

START WEIGHT:

END WEIGHT:

NUTRITIONAL INTAKE WRAP-UP

Did you meet your intake goals for the week? Why or why not?

_____
_____
_____
_____
_____
_____

DAYS I TRACKED MY DIET:

☐ Mon.
☐ Tues.
☐ Wed.
☐ Thurs.
☐ Fri.
☐ Sat.
☐ Sun.

EXERCISE WRAP-UP

Did you meet your exercise goals for the week? Why or why not?

_____
_____
_____
_____
_____

DAYS I EXERCISED:

☐ Mon.
☐ Tues.
☐ Wed.
☐ Thurs.
☐ Fri.
☐ Sat.
☐ Sun.

GOALS FOR NEXT WEEK

Things to work on for next week.

_____
_____
_____
_____
_____
_____
_____
_____

WEEKLY CALORIES BURNED:

WEEKLY ENERGY LEVEL:

☐ low
☐ medium
☐ high

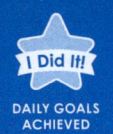

I Did It!
DAILY GOALS
ACHIEVED

MONDAY

DATE:

WEIGHT:

WATER INTAKE:
# of 8oz. glasses

☐ ☐ ☐ ☐
☐ ☐ ☐ ☐

ENERGY LEVEL:
☐ low
☐ medium
☐ high

DAILY # OF SERVINGS:

 fruits

 veggies

 grains

 meats & beans

 milk & dairy

 oils & sweets

VITAMINS & SUPPLEMENTS:

DAILY NUTRITIONAL INTAKE

Food/Beverages	Qty.	Calories	Fat	Carbs.	Protein	Fiber

DAILY TOTALS:

DAILY EXERCISE

Activity	Hrs./Mins.	Cal. Burned

DAILY TOTALS:

TIP OF THE DAY!

Work out because you want to. Make it the time of day when it's all about you.

DAILY NOTES, ACHIEVEMENTS

Obstacles, solutions, and thoughts on your progress.

TUESDAY

I Did It!

DAILY GOALS ACHIEVED

DAILY NUTRITIONAL INTAKE

Food/Beverages	Qty.	Calories	Fat	Carbs.	Protein	Fiber
_____	___					
_____	___					
_____	___					
_____	___					
_____	___					
_____	___					
_____	___					
_____	___					
_____	___					
_____	___					
_____	___					
_____	___					
_____	___					
_____	___					
_____	___					
DAILY TOTALS:						

DATE:

WEIGHT:

WATER INTAKE:
# of 8oz. glasses

☐ ☐ ☐ ☐
☐ ☐ ☐ ☐

ENERGY LEVEL:
☐ low
☐ medium
☐ high

DAILY # OF SERVINGS:

	fruits
	veggies
	grains
	meats & beans
	milk & dairy
	oils & sweets

VITAMINS & SUPPLEMENTS:
_____
_____
_____
_____
_____
_____

DAILY EXERCISE

Activity	Hrs./Mins.	Cal. Burned
_____	_____	
_____	_____	
_____	_____	
_____	_____	
_____	_____	
DAILY TOTALS:		

TIP OF THE DAY!

Stretch before and after you work out. Warming up your muscles is important to preventing injury.

DAILY NOTES, ACHIEVEMENTS

Obstacles, solutions, and thoughts on your progress.

_____
_____
_____

I Did It!

DAILY GOALS
ACHIEVED

WEEK
22

WEDNESDAY

DATE:

WEIGHT:

WATER INTAKE:
# of 8oz. glasses

☐ ☐ ☐ ☐
☐ ☐ ☐ ☐

ENERGY LEVEL:

☐ low
☐ medium
☐ high

DAILY # OF SERVINGS:

fruits

veggies

grains

meats & beans

milk & dairy

oils & sweets

VITAMINS & SUPPLEMENTS:

DAILY NUTRITIONAL INTAKE

Food/Beverages	Qty.	Calories	Fat	Carbs.	Protein	Fiber
DAILY TOTALS:						

DAILY EXERCISE

Activity	Hrs./Mins.	Cal. Burned
DAILY TOTALS:		

TIP OF THE DAY!

Stretching post-exercise helps you increase your flexibility and can decrease the possibility of soreness the next day.

DAILY NOTES, ACHIEVEMENTS

Obstacles, solutions, and thoughts on your progress.

THURSDAY

I Did It!

DAILY GOALS
ACHIEVED

DAILY NUTRITIONAL INTAKE

Food/Beverages	Qty.	Calories	Fat	Carbs.	Protein	Fiber
_____	___					
_____	___					
_____	___					
_____	___					
_____	___					
_____	___					
_____	___					
_____	___					
_____	___					
_____	___					
_____	___					
_____	___					
_____	___					
_____	___					
_____	___					
_____	___					
_____	___					
DAILY TOTALS:						

DATE:

WEIGHT:

WATER INTAKE:
# of 8oz. glasses
☐ ☐ ☐ ☐
☐ ☐ ☐ ☐

ENERGY LEVEL:
☐ low
☐ medium
☐ high

DAILY # OF SERVINGS:
fruits
veggies
grains
meats & beans
milk & dairy
oils & sweets

VITAMINS & SUPPLEMENTS:
_____
_____
_____
_____
_____

DAILY EXERCISE

Activity	Hrs./Mins.	Cal. Burned
_____	_____	
_____	_____	
_____	_____	
_____	_____	
_____	_____	
DAILY TOTALS:		

TIP OF THE DAY!

Identify and avoid the foods that send your appetite out of control. Common trigger foods usually combine sugar and fat, or fat and salt.

DAILY NOTES, ACHIEVEMENTS

Obstacles, solutions, and thoughts on your progress.

_____
_____
_____

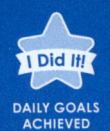

I Did It!

DAILY GOALS
ACHIEVED

DATE:

WEIGHT:

WATER INTAKE:
# of 8oz. glasses

☐ ☐ ☐ ☐
☐ ☐ ☐ ☐

ENERGY LEVEL:
☐ low
☐ medium
☐ high

DAILY # OF SERVINGS:

fruits

veggies

grains

meats & beans

milk & dairy

oils & sweets

VITAMINS & SUPPLEMENTS:

DAILY NUTRITIONAL INTAKE						
Food/Beverages	Qty.	Calories	Fat	Carbs.	Protein	Fiber
DAILY TOTALS:						

DAILY EXERCISE		
Activity	Hrs./Mins.	Cal. Burned
DAILY TOTALS:		

TIP OF THE DAY!

Take a day off from your workout every few days. This can prevent burnout, help you stay motivated and improve your results!

DAILY NOTES, ACHIEVEMENTS

Obstacles, solutions, and thoughts on your progress.

SATURDAY

I Did It!

DAILY GOALS
ACHIEVED

DAILY NUTRITIONAL INTAKE

Food/Beverages	Qty.	Calories	Fat	Carbs.	Protein	Fiber
DAILY TOTALS:						

DAILY EXERCISE

Activity	Hrs./Mins.	Cal. Burned
DAILY TOTALS:		

TIP OF THE DAY!

Before you begin eating, determine how much of the food on your plate you are going to eat. This will prevent you from overeating.

DAILY NOTES, ACHIEVEMENTS

Obstacles, solutions, and thoughts on your progress.

DATE:

WEIGHT:

WATER INTAKE:
# of 8oz. glasses

☐ ☐ ☐ ☐
☐ ☐ ☐ ☐

ENERGY LEVEL:
☐ low
☐ medium
☐ high

DAILY # OF SERVINGS:

fruits

veggies

grains

meats & beans

milk & dairy

oils & sweets

VITAMINS & SUPPLEMENTS:

I Did It!
DAILY GOALS ACHIEVED

WEEK
22

SUNDAY

DATE:

WEIGHT:

WATER INTAKE:
# of 8oz. glasses
☐ ☐ ☐ ☐
☐ ☐ ☐ ☐

ENERGY LEVEL:
☐ low
☐ medium
☐ high

DAILY # OF SERVINGS:

fruits

veggies

grains

meats & beans

milk & dairy

oils & sweets

VITAMINS & SUPPLEMENTS:

DAILY NUTRITIONAL INTAKE						
Food/Beverages	Qty.	Calories	Fat	Carbs.	Protein	Fiber
DAILY TOTALS:						

DAILY EXERCISE		
Activity	Hrs./Mins.	Cal. Burned
DAILY TOTALS:		

TIP OF THE DAY!

Don't eat if you're not hungry.

DAILY NOTES, ACHIEVEMENTS
Obstacles, solutions, and thoughts on your progress.

WEEKLY PROGRESS

WEEK 22

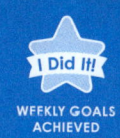

I Did It!

WEEKLY GOALS ACHIEVED

HIGHLIGHT OF THE WEEK

Your single-greatest moment of the week!

_____

_____

_____

_____

START WEIGHT:

END WEIGHT:

NUTRITIONAL INTAKE WRAP-UP

Did you meet your intake goals for the week? Why or why not?

_____

_____

_____

_____

_____

_____

DAYS I TRACKED MY DIET:

☐ Mon.
☐ Tues.
☐ Wed.
☐ Thurs.
☐ Fri.
☐ Sat.
☐ Sun.

EXERCISE WRAP-UP

Did you meet your exercise goals for the week? Why or why not?

_____

_____

_____

_____

_____

DAYS I EXERCISED:

☐ Mon.
☐ Tues.
☐ Wed.
☐ Thurs.
☐ Fri.
☐ Sat.
☐ Sun.

GOALS FOR NEXT WEEK

Things to work on for next week.

_____

_____

_____

_____

_____

_____

_____

_____

WEEKLY CALORIES BURNED:

WEEKLY ENERGY LEVEL:

☐ low
☐ medium
☐ high

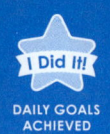
I Did It!
DAILY GOALS
ACHIEVED

MONDAY

DATE:

WEIGHT:

WATER INTAKE:
# of 8oz. glasses

☐ ☐ ☐ ☐
☐ ☐ ☐ ☐

ENERGY LEVEL:
☐ low
☐ medium
☐ high

DAILY # OF SERVINGS:

fruits

veggies

grains

meats & beans

milk & dairy

oils & sweets

VITAMINS & SUPPLEMENTS:

DAILY NUTRITIONAL INTAKE

Food/Beverages	Qty.	Calories	Fat	Carbs.	Protein	Fiber
DAILY TOTALS:						

DAILY EXERCISE

Activity	Hrs./Mins.	Cal. Burned
DAILY TOTALS:		

TIP OF THE DAY!

Take your weight-loss program one day at a time. Success is most often gradual, not instant.

DAILY NOTES, ACHIEVEMENTS
Obstacles, solutions, and thoughts on your progress.

TUESDAY

I Did It!

DAILY GOALS ACHIEVED

DAILY NUTRITIONAL INTAKE

Food/Beverages	Qty.	Calories	Fat	Carbs.	Protein	Fiber
_____						
_____						
_____						
_____						
_____						
_____						
_____						
_____						
_____						
_____						
_____						
_____						
_____						
_____						
_____						
_____						
_____						
DAILY TOTALS:						

DATE:

WEIGHT:

WATER INTAKE:
# of 8oz. glasses
☐ ☐ ☐ ☐
☐ ☐ ☐ ☐

ENERGY LEVEL:
☐ low
☐ medium
☐ high

DAILY # OF SERVINGS:

fruits

veggies

grains

meats & beans

milk & dairy

oils & sweets

VITAMINS & SUPPLEMENTS:

_____
_____
_____
_____
_____
_____
_____

DAILY EXERCISE

Activity	Hrs./Mins.	Cal. Burned
_____	_____	
_____	_____	
_____	_____	
_____	_____	
_____	_____	
DAILY TOTALS:		

TIP OF THE DAY!

Realize that seeing foods you crave can make you want to eat them more.

DAILY NOTES, ACHIEVEMENTS

Obstacles, solutions, and thoughts on your progress.

_____
_____
_____

I Did It!

DAILY GOALS ACHIEVED

WEEK 23 WEDNESDAY

DATE:

WEIGHT:

WATER INTAKE:
# of 8oz. glasses

☐ ☐ ☐ ☐
☐ ☐ ☐ ☐

ENERGY LEVEL:

☐ low
☐ medium
☐ high

DAILY # OF SERVINGS:

fruits

veggies

grains

meats & beans

milk & dairy

oils & sweets

VITAMINS & SUPPLEMENTS:

DAILY NUTRITIONAL INTAKE

Food/Beverages	Qty.	Calories	Fat	Carbs.	Protein	Fiber
DAILY TOTALS:						

DAILY EXERCISE

Activity	Hrs./Mins.	Cal. Burned
DAILY TOTALS:		

TIP OF THE DAY!

Add a little bit of sweetness to your main meal to prevent a craving for dessert.

DAILY NOTES, ACHIEVEMENTS

Obstacles, solutions, and thoughts on your progress.

THURSDAY

I Did It!

DAILY GOALS ACHIEVED

DAILY NUTRITIONAL INTAKE

Food/Beverages	Qty.	Calories	Fat	Carbs.	Protein	Fiber
DAILY TOTALS:						

DATE:

WEIGHT:

WATER INTAKE:
# of 8oz. glasses

☐ ☐ ☐ ☐
☐ ☐ ☐ ☐

ENERGY LEVEL:

☐ low

☐ medium

☐ high

DAILY # OF SERVINGS:

fruits

veggies

grains

meats & beans

milk & dairy

oils & sweets

VITAMINS & SUPPLEMENTS:

DAILY EXERCISE

Activity	Hrs./Mins.	Cal. Burned
DAILY TOTALS:		

TIP OF THE DAY!

Avoid alcohol: Drinking too much may decrease your ability to burn fat as well as reduce your willpower and self control.

DAILY NOTES, ACHIEVEMENTS

Obstacles, solutions, and thoughts on your progress.

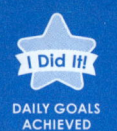

I Did It!

DAILY GOALS
ACHIEVED

WEEK
23

FRIDAY

DATE:

WEIGHT:

WATER INTAKE:
# of 8oz. glasses

☐ ☐ ☐ ☐
☐ ☐ ☐ ☐

ENERGY LEVEL:
☐ low
☐ medium
☐ high

DAILY # OF SERVINGS:

fruits

veggies

grains

meats & beans

milk & dairy

oils & sweets

VITAMINS & SUPPLEMENTS:

DAILY NUTRITIONAL INTAKE

Food/Beverages	Qty.	Calories	Fat	Carbs.	Protein	Fiber
DAILY TOTALS:						

DAILY EXERCISE

Activity	Hrs./Mins.	Cal. Burned
DAILY TOTALS:		

TIP OF THE DAY!

Skip large, heavy meals of white pasta, rice, bread, or pastries and donuts, which may make you feel hungry again within a short time.

DAILY NOTES, ACHIEVEMENTS

Obstacles, solutions, and thoughts on your progress.

SATURDAY

I Did It!

DAILY GOALS
ACHIEVED

DAILY NUTRITIONAL INTAKE

Food/Beverages	Qty.	Calories	Fat	Carbs.	Protein	Fiber
DAILY TOTALS:						

DAILY EXERCISE

Activity	Hrs./Mins.	Cal. Burned
DAILY TOTALS:		

TIP OF THE DAY!

Choose your diet plan carefully. You won't stick to a diet with foods you don't like, so choose a program that will include your favorite foods.

DAILY NOTES, ACHIEVEMENTS

Obstacles, solutions, and thoughts on your progress.

DATE:

WEIGHT:

WATER INTAKE:
# of 8oz. glasses

ENERGY LEVEL:
☐ low
☐ medium
☐ high

DAILY # OF SERVINGS:

fruits

veggies

grains

meats & beans

milk & dairy

oils & sweets

VITAMINS & SUPPLEMENTS:

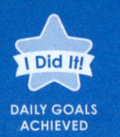

I Did It!

DAILY GOALS
ACHIEVED

DATE:

WEIGHT:

WATER INTAKE:
# of 8oz. glasses

☐ ☐ ☐ ☐
☐ ☐ ☐ ☐

ENERGY LEVEL:

☐ low
☐ medium
☐ high

**DAILY # OF
SERVINGS:**

fruits

veggies

grains

meats &
beans

milk &
dairy

oils &
sweets

**VITAMINS &
SUPPLEMENTS:**

DAILY NUTRITIONAL INTAKE

Food/Beverages	Qty.	Calories	Fat	Carbs.	Protein	Fiber
DAILY TOTALS:						

DAILY EXERCISE

Activity	Hrs./Mins.	Cal. Burned
DAILY TOTALS:		

TIP OF THE DAY!

Eating foods rich in soluble and insoluble fiber increases the feeling of fullness and slows the rate at which you digest your food.

DAILY NOTES, ACHIEVEMENTS

Obstacles, solutions, and thoughts on your progress.

WEEKLY PROGRESS

WEEK
23

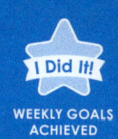

I Did It!

WEEKLY GOALS ACHIEVED

HIGHLIGHT OF THE WEEK

Your single-greatest moment of the week!

_____
_____
_____
_____

START WEIGHT:

END WEIGHT:

NUTRITIONAL INTAKE WRAP-UP

Did you meet your intake goals for the week? Why or why not?

_____
_____
_____
_____
_____
_____
_____

DAYS I TRACKED MY DIET:

☐ Mon.
☐ Tues.
☐ Wed.
☐ Thurs.
☐ Fri.
☐ Sat.
☐ Sun.

EXERCISE WRAP-UP

Did you meet your exercise goals for the week? Why or why not?

_____
_____
_____
_____
_____
_____

DAYS I EXERCISED:

☐ Mon.
☐ Tues.
☐ Wed.
☐ Thurs.
☐ Fri.
☐ Sat.
☐ Sun.

GOALS FOR NEXT WEEK

Things to work on for next week.

_____
_____
_____
_____
_____
_____
_____

WEEKLY CALORIES BURNED:

WEEKLY ENERGY LEVEL:

☐ low
☐ medium
☐ high

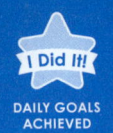

I Did It!
DAILY GOALS
ACHIEVED

WEEK
24

MONDAY

DATE:

WEIGHT:

WATER INTAKE:
# of 8oz. glasses
☐ ☐ ☐ ☐
☐ ☐ ☐ ☐

ENERGY LEVEL:
☐ low
☐ medium
☐ high

DAILY # OF SERVINGS:

fruits

veggies

grains

meats & beans

milk & dairy

oils & sweets

VITAMINS & SUPPLEMENTS:

DAILY NUTRITIONAL INTAKE

Food/Beverages	Qty.	Calories	Fat	Carbs.	Protein	Fiber
DAILY TOTALS:						

DAILY EXERCISE

Activity	Hrs./Mins.	Cal. Burned
DAILY TOTALS:		

TIP OF THE DAY!

Instead of dessert, choose a piece of fruit. Fruit can be more refreshing than sweets, and it will still satisfy your sweet tooth.

DAILY NOTES, ACHIEVEMENTS

Obstacles, solutions, and thoughts on your progress.

TUESDAY

24

I Did It!

DAILY GOALS ACHIEVED

DAILY NUTRITIONAL INTAKE

Food/Beverages	Qty.	Calories	Fat	Carbs.	Protein	Fiber
DAILY TOTALS:						

DATE:

WEIGHT:

WATER INTAKE:
# of 8oz. glasses
☐ ☐ ☐ ☐
☐ ☐ ☐ ☐

ENERGY LEVEL:
☐ low
☐ medium
☐ high

DAILY # OF SERVINGS:

fruits

veggies

grains

meats & beans

milk & dairy

oils & sweets

VITAMINS & SUPPLEMENTS:

DAILY EXERCISE

Activity	Hrs./Mins.	Cal. Burned
DAILY TOTALS:		

• TIP OF THE DAY!

Make healthy substitutions when cooking a meal. For example, you can use 2 egg whites instead of 1 egg, or replace the oil in a recipe with applesauce.

DAILY NOTES, ACHIEVEMENTS

Obstacles, solutions, and thoughts on your progress.

I Did It!
DAILY GOALS
ACHIEVED

DATE:

WEIGHT:

WATER INTAKE:
# of 8oz. glasses

☐ ☐ ☐ ☐
☐ ☐ ☐ ☐

ENERGY LEVEL:
☐ low
☐ medium
☐ high

DAILY # OF SERVINGS:

fruits

veggies

grains

meats & beans

milk & dairy

oils & sweets

VITAMINS & SUPPLEMENTS:

DAILY NUTRITIONAL INTAKE

Food/Beverages	Qty.	Calories	Fat	Carbs.	Protein	Fiber
DAILY TOTALS:						

DAILY EXERCISE

Activity	Hrs./Mins.	Cal. Burned
DAILY TOTALS:		

TIP OF THE DAY!

Brushing your teeth after meals can help curb your appetite.

DAILY NOTES, ACHIEVEMENTS

Obstacles, solutions, and thoughts on your progress.

THURSDAY

24

I Did It!

DAILY GOALS ACHIEVED

DAILY NUTRITIONAL INTAKE

Food/Beverages	Qty.	Calories	Fat	Carbs.	Protein	Fiber
DAILY TOTALS:						

DATE:

WEIGHT:

WATER INTAKE:
# of 8oz. glasses

☐ ☐ ☐ ☐
☐ ☐ ☐ ☐

ENERGY LEVEL:
☐ low
☐ medium
☐ high

DAILY # OF SERVINGS:

fruits

veggies

grains

meats & beans

milk & dairy

oils & sweets

VITAMINS & SUPPLEMENTS:

DAILY EXERCISE

Activity	Hrs./Mins.	Cal. Burned
DAILY TOTALS:		

TIP OF THE DAY!

Write down the reasons why you want to lose weight, and review them each week to maintain your motivation.

DAILY NOTES, ACHIEVEMENTS

Obstacles, solutions, and thoughts on your progress.

I Did It!
DAILY GOALS ACHIEVED

WEEK
24

FRIDAY

DATE:

WEIGHT:

WATER INTAKE:
# of 8oz. glasses

☐ ☐ ☐ ☐
☐ ☐ ☐ ☐

ENERGY LEVEL:
☐ low
☐ medium
☐ high

DAILY # OF SERVINGS:

fruits

veggies

grains

meats & beans

milk & dairy

oils & sweets

VITAMINS & SUPPLEMENTS:

DAILY NUTRITIONAL INTAKE

Food/Beverages	Qty.	Calories	Fat	Carbs.	Protein	Fiber
DAILY TOTALS:						

DAILY EXERCISE

Activity	Hrs./Mins.	Cal. Burned
DAILY TOTALS:		

TIP OF THE DAY!

Know that emotions such as boredom, happiness, or anxiety are causes of psychological hunger.

DAILY NOTES, ACHIEVEMENTS

Obstacles, solutions, and thoughts on your progress.

SATURDAY

I Did It!

DAILY GOALS
ACHIEVED

DAILY NUTRITIONAL INTAKE

Food/Beverages	Qty.	Calories	Fat	Carbs.	Protein	Fiber
DAILY TOTALS:						

DATE:

WEIGHT:

WATER INTAKE:
# of 8oz. glasses
☐ ☐ ☐ ☐
☐ ☐ ☐ ☐

ENERGY LEVEL:
☐ low
☐ medium
☐ high

DAILY # OF
SERVINGS:

fruits

veggies

grains

meats &
beans

milk &
dairy

oils &
sweets

VITAMINS &
SUPPLEMENTS:

DAILY EXERCISE

Activity	Hrs./Mins.	Cal. Burned
DAILY TOTALS:		

TIP OF THE DAY!

Let your friends and
family know that you
are dieting so they
can offer support
and encouragement.

DAILY NOTES, ACHIEVEMENTS

Obstacles, solutions, and thoughts on your progress.

I Did It!
DAILY GOALS ACHIEVED

SUNDAY

DATE:

WEIGHT:

WATER INTAKE:
# of 8oz. glasses
☐ ☐ ☐ ☐
☐ ☐ ☐ ☐

ENERGY LEVEL:
☐ low
☐ medium
☐ high

DAILY # OF SERVINGS:

fruits

veggies

grains

meats & beans

milk & dairy

oils & sweets

VITAMINS & SUPPLEMENTS:

DAILY NUTRITIONAL INTAKE

Food/Beverages	Qty.	Calories	Fat	Carbs.	Protein	Fiber
DAILY TOTALS:						

DAILY EXERCISE

Activity	Hrs./Mins.	Cal. Burned
DAILY TOTALS:		

TIP OF THE DAY!

Pass on snack mixes that combine a variety of chips, pretzels, and nuts. Too much variety can cause you to overeat.

DAILY NOTES, ACHIEVEMENTS

Obstacles, solutions, and thoughts on your progress.

WEEKLY PROGRESS

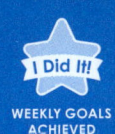

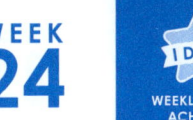
**WEEKLY GOALS
ACHIEVED**

HIGHLIGHT OF THE WEEK

Your single-greatest moment of the week!

_____
_____
_____
_____
_____

NUTRITIONAL INTAKE WRAP-UP

Did you meet your intake goals for the week? Why or why not?

_____
_____
_____
_____
_____
_____
_____

EXERCISE WRAP-UP

Did you meet your exercise goals for the week? Why or why not?

_____
_____
_____
_____
_____
_____

GOALS FOR NEXT WEEK

Things to work on for next week.

_____
_____
_____
_____
_____
_____
_____
_____
_____

START WEIGHT:

END WEIGHT:

DAYS I TRACKED MY DIET:
- ☐ Mon.
- ☐ Tues.
- ☐ Wed.
- ☐ Thurs.
- ☐ Fri.
- ☐ Sat.
- ☐ Sun.

DAYS I EXERCISED:
- ☐ Mon.
- ☐ Tues.
- ☐ Wed.
- ☐ Thurs.
- ☐ Fri.
- ☐ Sat.
- ☐ Sun.

WEEKLY CALORIES BURNED:

WEEKLY ENERGY LEVEL:
- ☐ low
- ☐ medium
- ☐ high

I Did It!

DAILY GOALS ACHIEVED

DATE:

WEIGHT:

WATER INTAKE:
# of 8oz. glasses

☐ ☐ ☐ ☐
☐ ☐ ☐ ☐

ENERGY LEVEL:
☐ low
☐ medium
☐ high

DAILY # OF SERVINGS:

fruits

veggies

grains

meats & beans

milk & dairy

oils & sweets

VITAMINS & SUPPLEMENTS:

DAILY NUTRITIONAL INTAKE

Food/Beverages	Qty.	Calories	Fat	Carbs.	Protein	Fiber
DAILY TOTALS:						

DAILY EXERCISE

Activity	Hrs./Mins.	Cal. Burned
DAILY TOTALS:		

TIP OF THE DAY!

Instead of coffee, try switching to green tea. Studies have shown a possible correlation between antioxidants found in green tea and overall good health.

DAILY NOTES, ACHIEVEMENTS

Obstacles, solutions, and thoughts on your progress.

TUESDAY

I Did It!

DAILY GOALS ACHIEVED

DAILY NUTRITIONAL INTAKE

Food/Beverages	Qty.	Calories	Fat	Carbs.	Protein	Fiber
_____	___					
_____	___					
_____	___					
_____	___					
_____	___					
_____	___					
_____	___					
_____	___					
_____	___					
_____	___					
_____	___					
_____	___					
_____	___					
_____	___					
_____	___					
_____	___					
_____	___					
DAILY TOTALS:						

DATE:

WEIGHT:

WATER INTAKE:
# of 8oz. glasses
☐ ☐ ☐ ☐
☐ ☐ ☐ ☐

ENERGY LEVEL:
☐ low
☐ medium
☐ high

DAILY # OF SERVINGS:
fruits
veggies
grains
meats & beans
milk & dairy
oils & sweets

VITAMINS & SUPPLEMENTS:

_____
_____
_____
_____
_____
_____
_____

DAILY EXERCISE

Activity	Hrs./Mins.	Cal. Burned
_____	_____	
_____	_____	
_____	_____	
_____	_____	
_____	_____	
DAILY TOTALS:		

TIP OF THE DAY!

If you must have a late-night snack, make it something sensible, like cereal or fruit.

DAILY NOTES, ACHIEVEMENTS

Obstacles, solutions, and thoughts on your progress.

_____
_____
_____

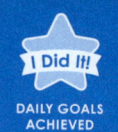

I Did It!

DAILY GOALS
ACHIEVED

WEEK
25

WEDNESDAY

DATE:

WEIGHT:

WATER INTAKE:
# of 8oz. glasses

☐ ☐ ☐ ☐
☐ ☐ ☐ ☐

ENERGY LEVEL:

☐ low
☐ medium
☐ high

**DAILY # OF
SERVINGS:**

fruits

veggies

grains

meats &
beans

milk &
dairy

oils &
sweets

**VITAMINS &
SUPPLEMENTS:**

DAILY NUTRITIONAL INTAKE

Food/Beverages	Qty.	Calories	Fat	Carbs.	Protein	Fiber
DAILY TOTALS:						

DAILY EXERCISE

Activity	Hrs./Mins.	Cal. Burned
DAILY TOTALS:		

TIP OF THE DAY!

Be the last person to
start eating when
dining with others.

DAILY NOTES, ACHIEVEMENTS

Obstacles, solutions, and thoughts on your progress.

THURSDAY

I Did It!
DAILY GOALS
ACHIEVED

DAILY NUTRITIONAL INTAKE

Food/Beverages	Qty.	Calories	Fat	Carbs.	Protein	Fiber
_____	____					
_____	____					
_____	____					
_____	____					
_____	____					
_____	____					
_____	____					
_____	____					
_____	____					
_____	____					
_____	____					
_____	____					
_____	____					
_____	____					
_____	____					
_____	____					
DAILY TOTALS:						

DATE:

WEIGHT:

WATER INTAKE:
# of 8oz. glasses
☐ ☐ ☐ ☐
☐ ☐ ☐ ☐

ENERGY LEVEL:
☐ low
☐ medium
☐ high

DAILY # OF SERVINGS:

	fruits
	veggies
	grains
	meats & beans
	milk & dairy
	oils & sweets

VITAMINS & SUPPLEMENTS:

_____
_____
_____
_____
_____
_____

DAILY EXERCISE

Activity	Hrs./Mins.	Cal. Burned
_____	____	
_____	____	
_____	____	
_____	____	
DAILY TOTALS:		

TIP OF THE DAY!

Before beginning an exercise routine, assess your health and physical status to ensure that you won't overexert or harm yourself.

DAILY NOTES, ACHIEVEMENTS

Obstacles, solutions, and thoughts on your progress.

_____
_____
_____

I Did It!

DAILY GOALS ACHIEVED

WEEK
25

FRIDAY

DATE:

WEIGHT:

WATER INTAKE:
# of 8oz. glasses

☐ ☐ ☐ ☐
☐ ☐ ☐ ☐

ENERGY LEVEL:
☐ low
☐ medium
☐ high

DAILY # OF SERVINGS:

fruits

veggies

grains

meats & beans

milk & dairy

oils & sweets

VITAMINS & SUPPLEMENTS:

DAILY NUTRITIONAL INTAKE						
Food/Beverages	Qty.	Calories	Fat	Carbs.	Protein	Fiber
DAILY TOTALS:						

DAILY EXERCISE		
Activity	Hrs./Mins.	Cal. Burned
DAILY TOTALS:		

TIP OF THE DAY!

Adopt a gradual approach to exercising, making a realistic plan for yourself.

DAILY NOTES, ACHIEVEMENTS
Obstacles, solutions, and thoughts on your progress.

SATURDAY

I Did It!

DAILY GOALS ACHIEVED

DAILY NUTRITIONAL INTAKE

Food/Beverages	Qty.	Calories	Fat	Carbs.	Protein	Fiber
DAILY TOTALS:						

DATE:

WEIGHT:

WATER INTAKE:
# of 8oz. glasses

☐ ☐ ☐ ☐
☐ ☐ ☐ ☐

ENERGY LEVEL:
☐ low
☐ medium
☐ high

DAILY # OF SERVINGS:

fruits

veggies

grains

meats & beans

milk & dairy

oils & sweets

VITAMINS & SUPPLEMENTS:

DAILY EXERCISE

Activity	Hrs./Mins.	Cal. Burned
DAILY TOTALS:		

TIP OF THE DAY!

Treating yourself to perks, such as a weekend getaway, massage, or new outfit, is a great way to celebrate your weight loss.

DAILY NOTES, ACHIEVEMENTS

Obstacles, solutions, and thoughts on your progress.

I Did It!

DAILY GOALS
ACHIEVED

WEEK
25

SUNDAY

DATE:

WEIGHT:

WATER INTAKE:
# of 8oz. glasses

☐ ☐ ☐ ☐
☐ ☐ ☐ ☐

ENERGY LEVEL:
☐ low
☐ medium
☐ high

DAILY # OF SERVINGS:

fruits

veggies

grains

meats & beans

milk & dairy

oils & sweets

VITAMINS & SUPPLEMENTS:

DAILY NUTRITIONAL INTAKE						
Food/Beverages	Qty.	Calories	Fat	Carbs.	Protein	Fiber
DAILY TOTALS:						

DAILY EXERCISE		
Activity	Hrs./Mins.	Cal. Burned
DAILY TOTALS:		

TIP OF THE DAY!

Cut calories and still eat your favorite foods by dividing your meal and only eating half. Substitute the other half with soup, fresh veggies, or a piece of fruit.

DAILY NOTES, ACHIEVEMENTS

Obstacles, solutions, and thoughts on your progress.

WEEKLY PROGRESS

WEEK 25

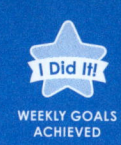

I Did It!

WEEKLY GOALS ACHIEVED

HIGHLIGHT OF THE WEEK

Your single-greatest moment of the week!

_____
_____
_____
_____
_____

START WEIGHT:

END WEIGHT:

NUTRITIONAL INTAKE WRAP-UP

Did you meet your intake goals for the week? Why or why not?

_____
_____
_____
_____
_____
_____

DAYS I TRACKED MY DIET:

- ☐ Mon.
- ☐ Tues.
- ☐ Wed.
- ☐ Thurs.
- ☐ Fri.
- ☐ Sat.
- ☐ Sun.

EXERCISE WRAP-UP

Did you meet your exercise goals for the week? Why or why not?

_____
_____
_____
_____
_____

DAYS I EXERCISED:

- ☐ Mon.
- ☐ Tues.
- ☐ Wed.
- ☐ Thurs.
- ☐ Fri.
- ☐ Sat.
- ☐ Sun.

GOALS FOR NEXT WEEK

Things to work on for next week.

_____
_____
_____
_____
_____
_____
_____

WEEKLY CALORIES BURNED:

WEEKLY ENERGY LEVEL:

- ☐ low
- ☐ medium
- ☐ high

MONTHLY

DATE:

START WEIGHT:

END WEIGHT:

BODY FAT %:

MEASUREMENTS:

chest

biceps

waist

hips

thighs

NOTES:

PHOTO OF THE MONTH

Photo comments.

tape your photo here

PROGRESS

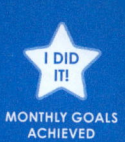

I DID IT!

MONTHLY GOALS ACHIEVED

HIGHLIGHT OF THE MONTH

Your single-greatest moment of the month!

_____
_____
_____
_____
_____

NUTRITIONAL INTAKE WRAP-UP

Did you meet your intake goals for the month? Why or why not?

_____
_____
_____
_____
_____
_____
_____
_____

EXERCISE WRAP-UP

Did you meet your exercise goals for the month? Why or why not?

_____
_____
_____
_____
_____

GOALS FOR NEXT MONTH

Things to work on for next month.

_____
_____
_____
_____
_____
_____
_____

I Did It!

DAILY GOALS ACHIEVED

WEEK
26

MONDAY

DATE:

WEIGHT:

WATER INTAKE:
# of 8oz. glasses

☐ ☐ ☐ ☐
☐ ☐ ☐ ☐

ENERGY LEVEL:

☐ low
☐ medium
☐ high

DAILY # OF SERVINGS:

- fruits
- veggies
- grains
- meats & beans
- milk & dairy
- oils & sweets

VITAMINS & SUPPLEMENTS:

DAILY NUTRITIONAL INTAKE

Food/Beverages	Qty.	Calories	Fat	Carbs.	Protein	Fiber
DAILY TOTALS:						

DAILY EXERCISE

Activity	Hrs./Mins.	Cal. Burned
DAILY TOTALS:		

TIP OF THE DAY!

Do not buy anything mega-, super-, or king-sized.

DAILY NOTES, ACHIEVEMENTS

Obstacles, solutions, and thoughts on your progress.

TUESDAY

I Did It!

DAILY GOALS ACHIEVED

DAILY NUTRITIONAL INTAKE

Food/Beverages	Qty.	Calories	Fat	Carbs.	Protein	Fiber
DAILY TOTALS:						

DAILY EXERCISE

Activity	Hrs./Mins.	Cal. Burned
DAILY TOTALS:		

TIP OF THE DAY!

Order single items rather than combo or meal deals.

DAILY NOTES, ACHIEVEMENTS

Obstacles, solutions, and thoughts on your progress.

_____
_____
_____
_____

DATE:

WEIGHT:

WATER INTAKE:
# of 8oz. glasses

☐ ☐ ☐ ☐
☐ ☐ ☐ ☐

ENERGY LEVEL:

☐ low
☐ medium
☐ high

DAILY # OF SERVINGS:

fruits

veggies

grains

meats & beans

milk & dairy

oils & sweets

VITAMINS & SUPPLEMENTS:

_____
_____
_____
_____
_____
_____
_____

I Did It!

DAILY GOALS
ACHIEVED

WEEK 26 WEDNESDAY

DATE:

WEIGHT:

WATER INTAKE:
# of 8oz. glasses

☐ ☐ ☐ ☐
☐ ☐ ☐ ☐

ENERGY LEVEL:

☐ low
☐ medium
☐ high

DAILY # OF SERVINGS:

fruits

veggies

grains

meats & beans

milk & dairy

oils & sweets

VITAMINS & SUPPLEMENTS:

DAILY NUTRITIONAL INTAKE

Food/Beverages	Qty.	Calories	Fat	Carbs.	Protein	Fiber
DAILY TOTALS:						

DAILY EXERCISE

Activity	Hrs./Mins.	Cal. Burned
DAILY TOTALS:		

TIP OF THE DAY!

Check the nutrition label for your favorite foods. If you have been eating much more than the standard, cut down your portions.

DAILY NOTES, ACHIEVEMENTS

Obstacles, solutions, and thoughts on your progress.

THURSDAY

I Did It!

DAILY GOALS ACHIEVED

DAILY NUTRITIONAL INTAKE

Food/Beverages	Qty.	Calories	Fat	Carbs.	Protein	Fiber
_____	____					
_____	____					
_____	____					
_____	____					
_____	____					
_____	____					
_____	____					
_____	____					
_____	____					
_____	____					
_____	____					
_____	____					
_____	____					
_____	____					
_____	____					
_____	____					
DAILY TOTALS:						

DATE:

WEIGHT:

WATER INTAKE:
# of 8oz. glasses

☐ ☐ ☐ ☐
☐ ☐ ☐ ☐

ENERGY LEVEL:
☐ low
☐ medium
☐ high

DAILY # OF SERVINGS:
fruits
veggies
grains
meats & beans
milk & dairy
oils & sweets

VITAMINS & SUPPLEMENTS:

DAILY EXERCISE

Activity	Hrs./Mins.	Cal. Burned
_____	_____	
_____	_____	
_____	_____	
_____	_____	
DAILY TOTALS:		

TIP OF THE DAY!

Learn to eyeball portion sizes.

DAILY NOTES, ACHIEVEMENTS

Obstacles, solutions, and thoughts on your progress.

_____
_____
_____
_____

I Did It!
DAILY GOALS
ACHIEVED

FRIDAY

DATE:

WEIGHT:

WATER INTAKE:
# of 8oz. glasses

☐ ☐ ☐ ☐
☐ ☐ ☐ ☐

ENERGY LEVEL:

☐ low
☐ medium
☐ high

DAILY # OF SERVINGS:

fruits

veggies

grains

meats & beans

milk & dairy

oils & sweets

VITAMINS & SUPPLEMENTS:

_____
_____
_____
_____
_____

DAILY NUTRITIONAL INTAKE

Food/Beverages	Qty.	Calories	Fat	Carbs.	Protein	Fiber
DAILY TOTALS:						

DAILY EXERCISE

Activity	Hrs./Mins.	Cal. Burned
DAILY TOTALS:		

TIP OF THE DAY!

Purchase favorite snack foods in 100-calorie packs and eat just one.

DAILY NOTES, ACHIEVEMENTS

Obstacles, solutions, and thoughts on your progress.

_____
_____
_____
_____

SATURDAY

I Did It!
DAILY GOALS
ACHIEVED

DAILY NUTRITIONAL INTAKE

Food/Beverages	Qty.	Calories	Fat	Carbs.	Protein	Fiber
DAILY TOTALS:						

DATE:

WEIGHT:

WATER INTAKE:
# of 8oz. glasses

☐ ☐ ☐ ☐
☐ ☐ ☐ ☐

ENERGY LEVEL:

☐ low
☐ medium
☐ high

DAILY # OF SERVINGS:

fruits

veggies

grains

meats & beans

milk & dairy

oils & sweets

VITAMINS & SUPPLEMENTS:

DAILY EXERCISE

Activity	Hrs./Mins.	Cal. Burned
DAILY TOTALS:		

TIP OF THE DAY!

Lose weight by splitting an entree with a friend. Most restaurant portions will satisfy 2 people.

DAILY NOTES, ACHIEVEMENTS

Obstacles, solutions, and thoughts on your progress.

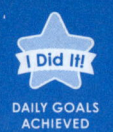

I Did It!
DAILY GOALS
ACHIEVED

WEEK
26

SUNDAY

DATE:

WEIGHT:

WATER INTAKE:
# of 8oz. glasses
☐ ☐ ☐ ☐
☐ ☐ ☐ ☐

ENERGY LEVEL:
☐ low
☐ medium
☐ high

DAILY # OF SERVINGS:

fruits

veggies

grains

meats & beans

milk & dairy

oils & sweets

VITAMINS & SUPPLEMENTS:

DAILY NUTRITIONAL INTAKE

Food/Beverages	Qty.	Calories	Fat	Carbs.	Protein	Fiber
DAILY TOTALS:						

DAILY EXERCISE

Activity	Hrs./Mins.	Cal. Burned
DAILY TOTALS:		

TIP OF THE DAY!

Ask your server to remove the bread basket when dining out.

DAILY NOTES, ACHIEVEMENTS

Obstacles, solutions, and thoughts on your progress.

WEEKLY PROGRESS

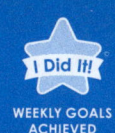

WEEKLY GOALS
ACHIEVED

HIGHLIGHT OF THE WEEK

Your single-greatest moment of the week!

_____
_____
_____
_____
_____

START WEIGHT:

END WEIGHT:

NUTRITIONAL INTAKE WRAP-UP

Did you meet your intake goals for the week? Why or why not?

_____
_____
_____
_____
_____
_____
_____

DAYS I TRACKED MY DIET:

☐ Mon.
☐ Tues.
☐ Wed.
☐ Thurs.
☐ Fri.
☐ Sat.
☐ Sun.

EXERCISE WRAP-UP

Did you meet your exercise goals for the week? Why or why not?

_____
_____
_____
_____
_____

DAYS I EXERCISED:

☐ Mon.
☐ Tues.
☐ Wed.
☐ Thurs.
☐ Fri.
☐ Sat.
☐ Sun.

GOALS FOR NEXT WEEK

Things to work on for next week.

_____
_____
_____
_____
_____
_____
_____

WEEKLY CALORIES BURNED:

WEEKLY ENERGY LEVEL:

☐ low
☐ medium
☐ high

I Did It!
DAILY GOALS ACHIEVED

MONDAY

DATE:

WEIGHT:

WATER INTAKE:
# of 8oz. glasses

☐ ☐ ☐ ☐
☐ ☐ ☐ ☐

ENERGY LEVEL:

☐ low
☐ medium
☐ high

DAILY # OF SERVINGS:

fruits

veggies

grains

meats & beans

milk & dairy

oils & sweets

VITAMINS & SUPPLEMENTS:

DAILY NUTRITIONAL INTAKE

Food/Beverages	Qty.	Calories	Fat	Carbs.	Protein	Fiber
DAILY TOTALS:						

DAILY EXERCISE

Activity	Hrs./Mins.	Cal. Burned
DAILY TOTALS:		

TIP OF THE DAY!

Don't be afraid to ask how something is prepared when dining out. If the preparation isn't in line with your diet plan, ask that it be made another way.

DAILY NOTES, ACHIEVEMENTS

Obstacles, solutions, and thoughts on your progress.

TUESDAY

I Did It!

DAILY GOALS
ACHIEVED

DAILY NUTRITIONAL INTAKE

Food/Beverages	Qty.	Calories	Fat	Carbs.	Protein	Fiber
DAILY TOTALS:						

DAILY EXERCISE

Activity	Hrs./Mins.	Cal. Burned
DAILY TOTALS:		

TIP OF THE DAY!

If you feel hungry again shortly after eating, ask yourself if something emotional, such as boredom or stress, is causing cravings, rather than real hunger.

DAILY NOTES, ACHIEVEMENTS

Obstacles, solutions, and thoughts on your progress.

DATE:

WEIGHT:

WATER INTAKE:

# of 8oz. glasses

☐ ☐ ☐ ☐
☐ ☐ ☐ ☐

ENERGY LEVEL:

☐ low
☐ medium
☐ high

DAILY # OF SERVINGS:

fruits

veggies

grains

meats & beans

milk & dairy

oils & sweets

VITAMINS & SUPPLEMENTS:

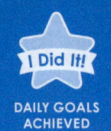

I Did It!

DAILY GOALS
ACHIEVED

DATE:

WEIGHT:

WATER INTAKE:
# of 8oz. glasses

☐ ☐ ☐ ☐
☐ ☐ ☐ ☐

ENERGY LEVEL:

☐ low
☐ medium
☐ high

DAILY # OF
SERVINGS:

fruits

veggies

grains

meats &
beans

milk &
dairy

oils &
sweets

VITAMINS &
SUPPLEMENTS:

DAILY NUTRITIONAL INTAKE

Food/Beverages	Qty.	Calories	Fat	Carbs.	Protein	Fiber
DAILY TOTALS:						

DAILY EXERCISE

Activity	Hrs./Mins.	Cal. Burned
DAILY TOTALS:		

TIP OF THE DAY!

When dining out,
order an appetizer
as your meal. Many
are large enough to
fill you up but not as
large as an entree.

DAILY NOTES, ACHIEVEMENTS

Obstacles, solutions, and thoughts on your progress.

THURSDAY

WEEK
27

I Did It!

**DAILY GOALS
ACHIEVED**

DAILY NUTRITIONAL INTAKE

Food/Beverages	Qty.	Calories	Fat	Carbs.	Protein	Fiber
DAILY TOTALS:						

DAILY EXERCISE

Activity	Hrs./Mins.	Cal. Burned
DAILY TOTALS:		

TIP OF THE DAY!

If someone at your workplace always has candy or snacks at his or her desk, be wary of mindless snacking.

DAILY NOTES, ACHIEVEMENTS

Obstacles, solutions, and thoughts on your progress.

DATE:

WEIGHT:

WATER INTAKE:
# of 8oz. glasses

☐ ☐ ☐ ☐
☐ ☐ ☐ ☐

ENERGY LEVEL:
☐ low
☐ medium
☐ high

DAILY # OF SERVINGS:

fruits

veggies

grains

meats & beans

milk & dairy

oils & sweets

VITAMINS & SUPPLEMENTS:

Journal Pages   265

I Did It!
DAILY GOALS
ACHIEVED

DATE:

WEIGHT:

WATER INTAKE:
# of 8oz. glasses
☐ ☐ ☐ ☐
☐ ☐ ☐ ☐

ENERGY LEVEL:
☐ low
☐ medium
☐ high

DAILY # OF SERVINGS:

fruits

veggies

grains

meats & beans

milk & dairy

oils & sweets

VITAMINS & SUPPLEMENTS:

DAILY NUTRITIONAL INTAKE

Food/Beverages	Qty.	Calories	Fat	Carbs.	Protein	Fiber
DAILY TOTALS:						

DAILY EXERCISE

Activity	Hrs./Mins.	Cal. Burned
DAILY TOTALS:		

TIP OF THE DAY!

At a party, avoid standing near the doorway to the kitchen where you will be the first person servers carrying fresh hors d'oeuvres will see.

DAILY NOTES, ACHIEVEMENTS

Obstacles, solutions, and thoughts on your progress.

SATURDAY

I Did It!

**DAILY GOALS
ACHIEVED**

DAILY NUTRITIONAL INTAKE

Food/Beverages	Qty.	Calories	Fat	Carbs.	Protein	Fiber
DAILY TOTALS:						

DAILY EXERCISE

Activity	Hrs./Mins.	Cal. Burned
DAILY TOTALS:		

TIP OF THE DAY!

At happy hour with coworkers or friends, order a seltzer water with lime instead of an alcoholic drink. Alcohol can whet the appetite.

DAILY NOTES, ACHIEVEMENTS

Obstacles, solutions, and thoughts on your progress.

DATE:

WEIGHT:

WATER INTAKE:
# of 8oz. glasses
☐ ☐ ☐ ☐
☐ ☐ ☐ ☐

ENERGY LEVEL:
☐ low
☐ medium
☐ high

DAILY # OF SERVINGS:
fruits
veggies
grains
meats & beans
milk & dairy
oils & sweets

VITAMINS & SUPPLEMENTS:

I Did It!

DAILY GOALS
ACHIEVED

DATE:

WEIGHT:

WATER INTAKE:
# of 8oz. glasses

☐ ☐ ☐ ☐
☐ ☐ ☐ ☐

ENERGY LEVEL:
☐ low
☐ medium
☐ high

DAILY # OF SERVINGS:

fruits

veggies

grains

meats & beans

milk & dairy

oils & sweets

VITAMINS & SUPPLEMENTS:

DAILY NUTRITIONAL INTAKE

Food/Beverages	Qty.	Calories	Fat	Carbs.	Protein	Fiber
DAILY TOTALS:						

DAILY EXERCISE

Activity	Hrs./Mins.	Cal. Burned
DAILY TOTALS:		

TIP OF THE DAY!

Don't add or remove anything from your frozen diet meals. These meals are designed to be nutritionally balanced and the right amount to fill you up.

DAILY NOTES, ACHIEVEMENTS

Obstacles, solutions, and thoughts on your progress.

WEEKLY PROGRESS

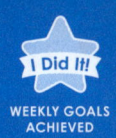

I Did It!

WEEKLY GOALS
ACHIEVED

HIGHLIGHT OF THE WEEK

Your single-greatest moment of the week!

_____

_____

_____

_____

START WEIGHT:

END WEIGHT:

NUTRITIONAL INTAKE WRAP-UP

Did you meet your intake goals for the week? Why or why not?

_____

_____

_____

_____

_____

_____

DAYS I TRACKED MY DIET:

☐ Mon.

☐ Tues.

☐ Wed.

☐ Thurs.

☐ Fri.

☐ Sat.

☐ Sun.

EXERCISE WRAP-UP

Did you meet your exercise goals for the week? Why or why not?

_____

_____

_____

_____

_____

DAYS I EXERCISED:

☐ Mon.

☐ Tues.

☐ Wed.

☐ Thurs.

☐ Fri.

☐ Sat.

☐ Sun.

GOALS FOR NEXT WEEK

Things to work on for next week.

_____

_____

_____

_____

_____

_____

_____

WEEKLY CALORIES BURNED:

WEEKLY ENERGY LEVEL:

☐ low

☐ medium

☐ high

I Did It!

DAILY GOALS
ACHIEVED

MONDAY

DATE:

WEIGHT:

WATER INTAKE:
# of 8oz. glasses

☐ ☐ ☐ ☐
☐ ☐ ☐ ☐

ENERGY LEVEL:
☐ low
☐ medium
☐ high

DAILY # OF
SERVINGS:

fruits

veggies

grains

meats &
beans

milk &
dairy

oils &
sweets

VITAMINS &
SUPPLEMENTS:

DAILY NUTRITIONAL INTAKE						
Food/Beverages	Qty.	Calories	Fat	Carbs.	Protein	Fiber
DAILY TOTALS:						

DAILY EXERCISE		
Activity	Hrs./Mins.	Cal. Burned
DAILY TOTALS:		

TIP OF THE DAY!

Low-fat, low-calorie dips like hummus are a nutritious way to spice up raw vegetables when you need a snack.

DAILY NOTES, ACHIEVEMENTS

Obstacles, solutions, and thoughts on your progress.

TUESDAY

I Did It!

**DAILY GOALS
ACHIEVED**

DAILY NUTRITIONAL INTAKE

Food/Beverages	Qty.	Calories	Fat	Carbs.	Protein	Fiber
_____	___					
_____	___					
_____	___					
_____	___					
_____	___					
_____	___					
_____	___					
_____	___					
_____	___					
_____	___					
_____	___					
_____	___					
_____	___					
_____	___					
_____	___					
_____	___					
_____	___					
DAILY TOTALS:						

DATE:

WEIGHT:

WATER INTAKE:
# of 8oz. glasses

☐ ☐ ☐ ☐
☐ ☐ ☐ ☐

ENERGY LEVEL:
☐ low
☐ medium
☐ high

**DAILY # OF
SERVINGS:**

fruits

veggies

grains

meats &
beans

milk &
dairy

oils &
sweets

**VITAMINS &
SUPPLEMENTS:**

DAILY EXERCISE

Activity	Hrs./Mins.	Cal. Burned
_____	_____	
_____	_____	
_____	_____	
_____	_____	
_____	_____	
DAILY TOTALS:		

TIP OF THE DAY!

If restaurant vegetables come in a separate side dish, this is a sign that they were cooked in oil and butter. Ask that they be steamed or roasted instead.

DAILY NOTES, ACHIEVEMENTS

Obstacles, solutions, and thoughts on your progress.

_____

_____

_____

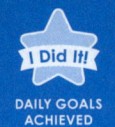

I Did It!
DAILY GOALS
ACHIEVED

WEEK
28

WEDNESDAY

DATE:

WEIGHT:

WATER INTAKE:
# of 8oz. glasses
☐ ☐ ☐ ☐
☐ ☐ ☐ ☐

ENERGY LEVEL:
☐ low
☐ medium
☐ high

DAILY # OF SERVINGS:

fruits

veggies

grains

meats & beans

milk & dairy

oils & sweets

VITAMINS & SUPPLEMENTS:

DAILY NUTRITIONAL INTAKE

Food/Beverages	Qty.	Calories	Fat	Carbs.	Protein	Fiber
DAILY TOTALS:						

DAILY EXERCISE

Activity	Hrs./Mins.	Cal. Burned
DAILY TOTALS:		

TIP OF THE DAY!

If you find that you eat or drink wine while cooking, chew a piece of peppermint gum to prevent snacking.

DAILY NOTES, ACHIEVEMENTS

Obstacles, solutions, and thoughts on your progress.

THURSDAY

I Did It!

**DAILY GOALS
ACHIEVED**

DAILY NUTRITIONAL INTAKE

Food/Beverages	Qty.	Calories	Fat	Carbs.	Protein	Fiber
_____	_____					
_____	_____					
_____	_____					
_____	_____					
_____	_____					
_____	_____					
_____	_____					
_____	_____					
_____	_____					
_____	_____					
_____	_____					
_____	_____					
_____	_____					
_____	_____					
_____	_____					
_____	_____					
DAILY TOTALS:						

DATE:

WEIGHT:

WATER INTAKE:
# of 8oz. glasses

☐ ☐ ☐ ☐
☐ ☐ ☐ ☐

ENERGY LEVEL:
☐ low
☐ medium
☐ high

DAILY # OF SERVINGS:

fruits

veggies

grains

meats & beans

milk & dairy

oils & sweets

VITAMINS & SUPPLEMENTS:

DAILY EXERCISE

Activity	Hrs./Mins.	Cal. Burned
_____	_____	
_____	_____	
_____	_____	
_____	_____	
DAILY TOTALS:		

TIP OF THE DAY!

Know that taking a supplement or multivitamin won't counteract an unhealthy diet or lifestyle.

DAILY NOTES, ACHIEVEMENTS

Obstacles, solutions, and thoughts on your progress.

_____

_____

_____

I Did It!
DAILY GOALS ACHIEVED

WEEK
28

FRIDAY

DATE:

WEIGHT:

WATER INTAKE:
# of 8oz. glasses

☐ ☐ ☐ ☐
☐ ☐ ☐ ☐

ENERGY LEVEL:
☐ low
☐ medium
☐ high

DAILY # OF SERVINGS:

fruits

veggies

grains

meats & beans

milk & dairy

oils & sweets

VITAMINS & SUPPLEMENTS:

DAILY NUTRITIONAL INTAKE

Food/Beverages	Qty.	Calories	Fat	Carbs.	Protein	Fiber
DAILY TOTALS:						

DAILY EXERCISE

Activity	Hrs./Mins.	Cal. Burned
DAILY TOTALS:		

TIP OF THE DAY!

Beware of low-fat products. Studies have shown that dieters tend to eat more of products labeled as low fat.

DAILY NOTES, ACHIEVEMENTS

Obstacles, solutions, and thoughts on your progress.

SATURDAY

I Did It!

DAILY GOALS ACHIEVED

DAILY NUTRITIONAL INTAKE

Food/Beverages	Qty.	Calories	Fat	Carbs.	Protein	Fiber
DAILY TOTALS:						

DATE:

WEIGHT:

WATER INTAKE:
# of 8oz. glasses
☐ ☐ ☐ ☐
☐ ☐ ☐ ☐

ENERGY LEVEL:
☐ low
☐ medium
☐ high

DAILY # OF SERVINGS:
fruits
veggies
grains
meats & beans
milk & dairy
oils & sweets

VITAMINS & SUPPLEMENTS:

DAILY EXERCISE

Activity	Hrs./Mins.	Cal. Burned
DAILY TOTALS:		

TIP OF THE DAY!

If you don't like the taste of water, add lemons, limes, cucumber or orange slices to a pitcher to add flavor.

DAILY NOTES, ACHIEVEMENTS

Obstacles, solutions, and thoughts on your progress.

I Did It!

DAILY GOALS ACHIEVED

DATE:

WEIGHT:

WATER INTAKE:
# of 8oz. glasses

☐ ☐ ☐ ☐
☐ ☐ ☐ ☐

ENERGY LEVEL:

☐ low
☐ medium
☐ high

DAILY # OF SERVINGS:

fruits

veggies

grains

meats & beans

milk & dairy

oils & sweets

VITAMINS & SUPPLEMENTS:

DAILY NUTRITIONAL INTAKE

Food/Beverages	Qty.	Calories	Fat	Carbs.	Protein	Fiber
DAILY TOTALS:						

DAILY EXERCISE

Activity	Hrs./Mins.	Cal. Burned
DAILY TOTALS:		

TIP OF THE DAY!

Greek yogurt is an excellent substitute for sour cream and mayo in recipes like dips. It adds creamy texture without extra fat.

DAILY NOTES, ACHIEVEMENTS

Obstacles, solutions, and thoughts on your progress.

WEEKLY PROGRESS

WEEK
28

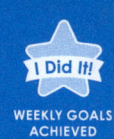

I Did It!

WEEKLY GOALS ACHIEVED

HIGHLIGHT OF THE WEEK

Your single-greatest moment of the week!

_____
_____
_____
_____

START WEIGHT:

END WEIGHT:

NUTRITIONAL INTAKE WRAP-UP

Did you meet your intake goals for the week? Why or why not?

_____
_____
_____
_____
_____
_____

DAYS I TRACKED MY DIET:

- ☐ Mon.
- ☐ Tues.
- ☐ Wed.
- ☐ Thurs.
- ☐ Fri.
- ☐ Sat.
- ☐ Sun.

EXERCISE WRAP-UP

Did you meet your exercise goals for the week? Why or why not?

_____
_____
_____
_____
_____

DAYS I EXERCISED:

- ☐ Mon.
- ☐ Tues.
- ☐ Wed.
- ☐ Thurs.
- ☐ Fri.
- ☐ Sat.
- ☐ Sun.

GOALS FOR NEXT WEEK

Things to work on for next week.

_____
_____
_____
_____
_____
_____
_____

WEEKLY CALORIES BURNED:

WEEKLY ENERGY LEVEL:

- ☐ low
- ☐ medium
- ☐ high

I Did It!

DAILY GOALS ACHIEVED

WEEK 29

MONDAY

DATE:

WEIGHT:

WATER INTAKE:
# of 8oz. glasses

☐ ☐ ☐ ☐
☐ ☐ ☐ ☐

ENERGY LEVEL:

☐ low
☐ medium
☐ high

DAILY # OF SERVINGS:

fruits

veggies

grains

meats & beans

milk & dairy

oils & sweets

VITAMINS & SUPPLEMENTS:

DAILY NUTRITIONAL INTAKE

Food/Beverages	Qty.	Calories	Fat	Carbs.	Protein	Fiber
DAILY TOTALS:						

DAILY EXERCISE

Activity	Hrs./Mins.	Cal. Burned
DAILY TOTALS:		

TIP OF THE DAY!

Instead of adding sugar to your coffee, sprinkle it with cinnamon for flavor without calories or carbs.

DAILY NOTES, ACHIEVEMENTS

Obstacles, solutions, and thoughts on your progress.

TUESDAY

I Did It!

DAILY GOALS ACHIEVED

DAILY NUTRITIONAL INTAKE

Food/Beverages	Qty.	Calories	Fat	Carbs.	Protein	Fiber
_____	___					
_____	___					
_____	___					
_____	___					
_____	___					
_____	___					
_____	___					
_____	___					
_____	___					
_____	___					
_____	___					
_____	___					
_____	___					
_____	___					
_____	___					
_____	___					
_____	___					
DAILY TOTALS:						

DATE:

WEIGHT:

WATER INTAKE:
# of 8oz. glasses
☐ ☐ ☐ ☐
☐ ☐ ☐ ☐

ENERGY LEVEL:
☐ low
☐ medium
☐ high

DAILY # OF SERVINGS:
fruits
veggies
grains
meats & beans
milk & dairy
oils & sweets

VITAMINS & SUPPLEMENTS:
_____
_____
_____
_____
_____
_____

DAILY EXERCISE

Activity	Hrs./Mins.	Cal. Burned
_____	_____	
_____	_____	
_____	_____	
_____	_____	
_____	_____	
DAILY TOTALS:		

TIP OF THE DAY!

Learn to eyeball proper portions by washing and saving the empty containers from frozen diet meals.

DAILY NOTES, ACHIEVEMENTS

Obstacles, solutions, and thoughts on your progress.

_____

_____

_____

I Did It!
DAILY GOALS ACHIEVED

WEEK
29

WEDNESDAY

DATE:

WEIGHT:

WATER INTAKE:
# of 8oz. glasses

☐ ☐ ☐ ☐
☐ ☐ ☐ ☐

ENERGY LEVEL:

☐ low
☐ medium
☐ high

DAILY # OF SERVINGS:

fruits

veggies

grains

meats & beans

milk & dairy

oils & sweets

VITAMINS & SUPPLEMENTS:

DAILY NUTRITIONAL INTAKE						
Food/Beverages	Qty.	Calories	Fat	Carbs.	Protein	Fiber
DAILY TOTALS:						

DAILY EXERCISE		
Activity	Hrs./Mins.	Cal. Burned
DAILY TOTALS:		

TIP OF THE DAY!

Writing down everything you eat and drink throughout the day can double your weight loss.

DAILY NOTES, ACHIEVEMENTS

Obstacles, solutions, and thoughts on your progress.

THURSDAY

I Did It!

DAILY GOALS
ACHIEVED

DAILY NUTRITIONAL INTAKE

Food/Beverages	Qty.	Calories	Fat	Carbs.	Protein	Fiber
_____	_____					
_____	_____					
_____	_____					
_____	_____					
_____	_____					
_____	_____					
_____	_____					
_____	_____					
_____	_____					
_____	_____					
_____	_____					
_____	_____					
_____	_____					
_____	_____					
_____	_____					
_____	_____					
_____	_____					
DAILY TOTALS:						

DATE:

WEIGHT:

WATER INTAKE:
# of 8oz. glasses

☐ ☐ ☐ ☐
☐ ☐ ☐ ☐

ENERGY LEVEL:

☐ low
☐ medium
☐ high

DAILY # OF SERVINGS:

fruits

veggies

grains

meats & beans

milk & dairy

oils & sweets

DAILY EXERCISE

Activity	Hrs./Mins.	Cal. Burned
_____	_____	
_____	_____	
_____	_____	
_____	_____	
_____	_____	
DAILY TOTALS:		

TIP OF THE DAY!

"Organic" doesn't indicate a food is healthy. Studies have shown that organic products have no more nutritional value than regular products.

VITAMINS & SUPPLEMENTS:

_____
_____
_____
_____
_____
_____
_____

DAILY NOTES, ACHIEVEMENTS

Obstacles, solutions, and thoughts on your progress.

_____
_____
_____

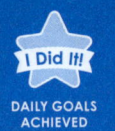

I Did It!
DAILY GOALS
ACHIEVED

FRIDAY

DATE:

WEIGHT:

WATER INTAKE:
# of 8oz. glasses

☐ ☐ ☐ ☐
☐ ☐ ☐ ☐

ENERGY LEVEL:

☐ low
☐ medium
☐ high

DAILY # OF SERVINGS:

fruits

veggies

grains

meats & beans

milk & dairy

oils & sweets

VITAMINS & SUPPLEMENTS:

DAILY NUTRITIONAL INTAKE

Food/Beverages	Qty.	Calories	Fat	Carbs.	Protein	Fiber
DAILY TOTALS:						

DAILY EXERCISE

Activity	Hrs./Mins.	Cal. Burned
DAILY TOTALS:		

TIP OF THE DAY!

Be conscious of how much you eat when dining out with friends. Women tend to eat much more in a group of women than when eating with men.

DAILY NOTES, ACHIEVEMENTS

Obstacles, solutions, and thoughts on your progress.

SATURDAY

I Did It!

DAILY GOALS
ACHIEVED

DAILY NUTRITIONAL INTAKE

Food/Beverages	Qty.	Calories	Fat	Carbs.	Protein	Fiber
DAILY TOTALS:						

DAILY EXERCISE

Activity	Hrs./Mins.	Cal. Burned
DAILY TOTALS:		

TIP OF THE DAY!

Some research has shown that diet soda actually makes people crave sugar. Switch to sparkling water instead.

DAILY NOTES, ACHIEVEMENTS

Obstacles, solutions, and thoughts on your progress.

DATE:

WEIGHT:

WATER INTAKE:
# of 8oz. glasses

☐ ☐ ☐ ☐
☐ ☐ ☐ ☐

ENERGY LEVEL:
☐ low
☐ medium
☐ high

DAILY # OF SERVINGS:

fruits

veggies

grains

meats & beans

milk & dairy

oils & sweets

VITAMINS & SUPPLEMENTS:

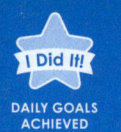

I Did It!
DAILY GOALS
ACHIEVED

WEEK
29

SUNDAY

DATE:

WEIGHT:

WATER INTAKE:
# of 8oz. glasses
☐ ☐ ☐ ☐
☐ ☐ ☐ ☐

ENERGY LEVEL:
☐ low
☐ medium
☐ high

DAILY # OF SERVINGS:

fruits

veggies

grains

meats & beans

milk & dairy

oils & sweets

VITAMINS & SUPPLEMENTS:

DAILY NUTRITIONAL INTAKE						
Food/Beverages	Qty.	Calories	Fat	Carbs.	Protein	Fiber
DAILY TOTALS:						

DAILY EXERCISE		
Activity	Hrs./Mins.	Cal. Burned
DAILY TOTALS:		

TIP OF THE DAY!

At a restaurant, order salad dressing on the side; then dip your fork into the dressing several times and spread it over the salad.

DAILY NOTES, ACHIEVEMENTS

Obstacles, solutions, and thoughts on your progress.

WEEKLY PROGRESS

WEEK 29

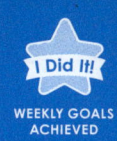

I Did It!

WEEKLY GOALS
ACHIEVED

HIGHLIGHT OF THE WEEK

Your single-greatest moment of the week!

_____

_____

_____

_____

NUTRITIONAL INTAKE WRAP-UP

Did you meet your intake goals for the week? Why or why not?

_____

_____

_____

_____

_____

_____

EXERCISE WRAP-UP

Did you meet your exercise goals for the week? Why or why not?

_____

_____

_____

_____

GOALS FOR NEXT WEEK

Things to work on for next week.

_____

_____

_____

_____

_____

_____

_____

START WEIGHT:

END WEIGHT:

DAYS I TRACKED MY DIET:
- ☐ Mon.
- ☐ Tues.
- ☐ Wed.
- ☐ Thurs.
- ☐ Fri.
- ☐ Sat.
- ☐ Sun.

DAYS I EXERCISED:
- ☐ Mon.
- ☐ Tues.
- ☐ Wed.
- ☐ Thurs.
- ☐ Fri.
- ☐ Sat.
- ☐ Sun.

WEEKLY CALORIES BURNED:

WEEKLY ENERGY LEVEL:
- ☐ low
- ☐ medium
- ☐ high

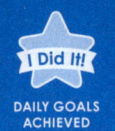

I Did It!
DAILY GOALS
ACHIEVED

MONDAY

DATE:

WEIGHT:

WATER INTAKE:
# of 8oz. glasses

☐ ☐ ☐ ☐
☐ ☐ ☐ ☐

ENERGY LEVEL:
☐ low
☐ medium
☐ high

DAILY # OF SERVINGS:

fruits

veggies

grains

meats & beans

milk & dairy

oils & sweets

VITAMINS & SUPPLEMENTS:

DAILY NUTRITIONAL INTAKE

Food/Beverages	Qty.	Calories	Fat	Carbs.	Protein	Fiber
DAILY TOTALS:						

DAILY EXERCISE

Activity	Hrs./Mins.	Cal. Burned
DAILY TOTALS:		

TIP OF THE DAY!

At a party, avoid dips that are full of fat and calories, including crab dip, spinach and artichoke dip, cheese dip, and onion dip.

DAILY NOTES, ACHIEVEMENTS

Obstacles, solutions, and thoughts on your progress.

TUESDAY

I Did It!

DAILY GOALS
ACHIEVED

DAILY NUTRITIONAL INTAKE

Food/Beverages	Qty.	Calories	Fat	Carbs.	Protein	Fiber
DAILY TOTALS:						

DATE:

WEIGHT:

WATER INTAKE:
# of 8oz. glasses
☐ ☐ ☐ ☐
☐ ☐ ☐ ☐

ENERGY LEVEL:
☐ low
☐ medium
☐ high

DAILY # OF SERVINGS:
fruits
veggies
grains
meats & beans
milk & dairy
oils & sweets

VITAMINS & SUPPLEMENTS:

DAILY EXERCISE

Activity	Hrs./Mins.	Cal. Burned
DAILY TOTALS:		

TIP OF THE DAY!

Don't let what others are eating affect what you order when dining out.

DAILY NOTES, ACHIEVEMENTS

Obstacles, solutions, and thoughts on your progress.

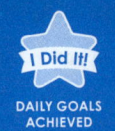

I Did It!

DAILY GOALS ACHIEVED

WEEK 30 **WEDNESDAY**

DATE:

WEIGHT:

WATER INTAKE:
# of 8oz. glasses

☐ ☐ ☐ ☐
☐ ☐ ☐ ☐

ENERGY LEVEL:

☐ low
☐ medium
☐ high

DAILY # OF SERVINGS:

fruits

veggies

grains

meats & beans

milk & dairy

oils & sweets

VITAMINS & SUPPLEMENTS:

DAILY NUTRITIONAL INTAKE

Food/Beverages	Qty.	Calories	Fat	Carbs.	Protein	Fiber
DAILY TOTALS:						

DAILY EXERCISE

Activity	Hrs./Mins.	Cal. Burned
DAILY TOTALS:		

TIP OF THE DAY!

Working out first thing in the morning can help jumpstart metabolism.

DAILY NOTES, ACHIEVEMENTS

Obstacles, solutions, and thoughts on your progress.

THURSDAY

I Did It!

DAILY GOALS ACHIEVED

DAILY NUTRITIONAL INTAKE

Food/Beverages	Qty.	Calories	Fat	Carbs.	Protein	Fiber
_____	____					
_____	____					
_____	____					
_____	____					
_____	____					
_____	____					
_____	____					
_____	____					
_____	____					
_____	____					
_____	____					
_____	____					
_____	____					
_____	____					
_____	____					
_____	____					
DAILY TOTALS:						

DATE:

WEIGHT:

WATER INTAKE:
# of 8oz. glasses

☐ ☐ ☐ ☐
☐ ☐ ☐ ☐

ENERGY LEVEL:
☐ low
☐ medium
☐ high

DAILY # OF SERVINGS:

fruits

veggies

grains

meats & beans

milk & dairy

oils & sweets

VITAMINS & SUPPLEMENTS:

_____
_____
_____
_____
_____
_____
_____

DAILY EXERCISE

Activity	Hrs./Mins.	Cal. Burned
_____	_____	
_____	_____	
_____	_____	
_____	_____	
_____	_____	
DAILY TOTALS:		

TIP OF THE DAY!

Smoothies sound healthy but beware of those made with ice cream or heavy cream.

DAILY NOTES, ACHIEVEMENTS

Obstacles, solutions, and thoughts on your progress.

_____
_____

I Did It!

DAILY GOALS
ACHIEVED

WEEK
30

FRIDAY

DATE:

WEIGHT:

WATER INTAKE:
# of 8oz. glasses

☐ ☐ ☐ ☐
☐ ☐ ☐ ☐

ENERGY LEVEL:

☐ low
☐ medium
☐ high

DAILY # OF SERVINGS:

fruits

veggies

grains

meats & beans

milk & dairy

oils & sweets

VITAMINS & SUPPLEMENTS:

DAILY NUTRITIONAL INTAKE						
Food/Beverages	Qty.	Calories	Fat	Carbs.	Protein	Fiber
DAILY TOTALS:						

DAILY EXERCISE		
Activity	Hrs./Mins.	Cal. Burned
DAILY TOTALS:		

TIP OF THE DAY!

There is no need to taste food again and again while cooking. Ask a family member to help you decide if something needs more spice.

DAILY NOTES, ACHIEVEMENTS

Obstacles, solutions, and thoughts on your progress.

SATURDAY

I Did It!

DAILY GOALS
ACHIEVED

DAILY NUTRITIONAL INTAKE

Food/Beverages	Qty.	Calories	Fat	Carbs.	Protein	Fiber
_____	_____					
_____	_____					
_____	_____					
_____	_____					
_____	_____					
_____	_____					
_____	_____					
_____	_____					
_____	_____					
_____	_____					
_____	_____					
_____	_____					
_____	_____					
_____	_____					
_____	_____					
_____	_____					
_____	_____					
DAILY TOTALS:						

DATE:

WEIGHT:

WATER INTAKE:
# of 8oz. glasses
☐ ☐ ☐ ☐
☐ ☐ ☐ ☐

ENERGY LEVEL:
☐ low
☐ medium
☐ high

DAILY # OF SERVINGS:
- fruits
- veggies
- grains
- meats & beans
- milk & dairy
- oils & sweets

VITAMINS & SUPPLEMENTS:
_____
_____
_____
_____
_____
_____

DAILY EXERCISE

Activity	Hrs./Mins.	Cal. Burned
_____	_____	
_____	_____	
_____	_____	
_____	_____	
_____	_____	
DAILY TOTALS:		

TIP OF THE DAY!

Don't cut calories here only to spend them there. If you order a light salad, don't drink a high-calorie margarita as well.

DAILY NOTES, ACHIEVEMENTS

Obstacles, solutions, and thoughts on your progress.

_____
_____
_____

I Did It!

DAILY GOALS
ACHIEVED

WEEK
30

SUNDAY

DATE:

WEIGHT:

WATER INTAKE:
# of 8oz. glasses

☐ ☐ ☐ ☐
☐ ☐ ☐ ☐

ENERGY LEVEL:

☐ low
☐ medium
☐ high

DAILY # OF SERVINGS:

fruits

veggies

grains

meats & beans

milk & dairy

oils & sweets

VITAMINS & SUPPLEMENTS:

DAILY NUTRITIONAL INTAKE

Food/Beverages	Qty.	Calories	Fat	Carbs.	Protein	Fiber
DAILY TOTALS:						

DAILY EXERCISE

Activity	Hrs./Mins.	Cal. Burned
DAILY TOTALS:		

TIP OF THE DAY!

Be honest with yourself about everything you eat when you write in your journal. Don't let even a handful of chips or a bite of a cookie slip by!

DAILY NOTES, ACHIEVEMENTS

Obstacles, solutions, and thoughts on your progress.

WEEKLY PROGRESS

WEEK 30

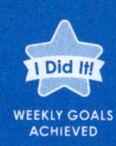

I Did It!

WEEKLY GOALS ACHIEVED

HIGHLIGHT OF THE WEEK

Your single-greatest moment of the week!

_____
_____
_____
_____

NUTRITIONAL INTAKE WRAP-UP

Did you meet your intake goals for the week? Why or why not?

_____
_____
_____
_____
_____
_____
_____

EXERCISE WRAP-UP

Did you meet your exercise goals for the week? Why or why not?

_____
_____
_____
_____
_____

GOALS FOR NEXT WEEK

Things to work on for next week.

_____
_____
_____
_____
_____
_____
_____
_____

START WEIGHT:

END WEIGHT:

DAYS I TRACKED MY DIET:
- [ ] Mon.
- [ ] Tues.
- [ ] Wed.
- [ ] Thurs.
- [ ] Fri.
- [ ] Sat.
- [ ] Sun.

DAYS I EXERCISED:
- [ ] Mon.
- [ ] Tues.
- [ ] Wed.
- [ ] Thurs.
- [ ] Fri.
- [ ] Sat.
- [ ] Sun.

WEEKLY CALORIES BURNED:

WEEKLY ENERGY LEVEL:
- [ ] low
- [ ] medium
- [ ] high

MONTHLY

DATE:

START WEIGHT:

END WEIGHT:

BODY FAT %:

MEASUREMENTS:

chest

biceps

waist

hips

thighs

NOTES:

PHOTO OF THE MONTH

Photo comments.

tape your photo here

PROGRESS

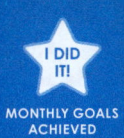

I DID IT!

MONTHLY GOALS ACHIEVED

HIGHLIGHT OF THE MONTH

Your single-greatest moment of the month!

_____

_____

_____

_____

NUTRITIONAL INTAKE WRAP-UP

Did you meet your intake goals for the month? Why or why not?

_____

_____

_____

_____

_____

_____

_____

EXERCISE WRAP-UP

Did you meet your exercise goals for the month? Why or why not?

_____

_____

_____

_____

GOALS FOR NEXT MONTH

Things to work on for next month.

_____

_____

_____

_____

_____

_____

NUTRITION FACTS

This section is a great resource for nutritional information on foods you may want to select for your weight-loss program. It provides calories per serving, as well as the content in grams for protein, and fats, carbohydrates, and fiber.

To use this section, look up a food item and its corresponding information. Then, log this data in your journal so that you can track your daily totals.

A helpful exercise is to make a list of all the foods you like that fit within your diet program so you can easily plan meals and go grocery shopping. Use the following chart to list those items:

COMMON ITEMS YOU LIKE TO EAT						
Food/Beverages	Qty.	Calories	Fat	Carbs.	Protein	Fiber

NUTRITION FACTS

FOOD ITEM	SERVING SIZE	CAL	FAT	PRTN	CBS	FBR
A						
Alcohol, 100 proof	1 fl.oz.	82	0	0	0	0
Alcohol, 86 proof	1 fl.oz.	70	0	0	0	0
Alcohol, 90 proof	1 fl.oz.	73	0	0	0	0
Alcohol, 94 proof	1 fl.oz.	76	0	0	0	0
Alcohol, dessert wine, dry	1 glass	157	0	0	12	0
Alcohol, dessert wine, sweet	1 glass	165	0	0	14	0
Alcohol, liquors	1 fl.oz.	107	0	0	11	0
Alcohol, pina colada	8 fl.oz.	440	5	1	57	0
Alfalfa seeds	1 tbsp	1	0	0	0	0
Allspice, ground	1 tsp	5	0	0	1	0
Almond butter, w/ salt	1 tbsp	101	10	2	3	1
Almond butter, w/o salt	1 tbsp	101	10	2	3	1
Almonds, roasted	1 oz. (12 nuts)	169	15	6	6	3
Anchovies	3 oz.	111	4	17	0	0
Apple cider, powdered	1 packet	83	0	0	21	0
Apple juice	8 fl.oz.	120	0	0	29	0
Apples, w/o skin	1 medium	61	0	0	16	2
Apples, w/ skin	1 medium	72	0	0	19	3
Applesauce	1 cup	194	1	1	51	3
Apricots	1 apricot	17	0	1	4	1
Arrowroot	1 cup, sliced	78	0	5	16	2
Arrowroot flour	1 cup	457	0	0	113	4
Artichokes	1 artichoke	76	0	5	17	9
Arugula	1 cup	4	0	1	1	0
Asparagus	1 spear	2	0	0	1	0
Avocados	1 cup, cubes	240	22	3	13	10
B						
Bacon bits, meatless	1 tbsp	33	2	2	2	1
Bacon, canadian, cooked	1 slice	43	2	6	0	0
Bacon, meatless	1 slice	16	2	1	0	0
Bacon, pork, cooked	1 slice	42	3	3	0	0
Bagels, cinnamon-raisin	1 bagel, 4" dia	244	2	9	49	2
Bagels, egg	1 bagel, 4" dia	292	2	11	56	2
Bagels, oat-bran	1 bagel, 4" dia	227	1	10	47	3
Bagels, plain	1 bagel, 4" dia	245	1	9	47	2
Bagels, deli gourmet style	1 bagel	370	3	13	71	2
Balsam pear	1 balsam pear	21	0	1	5	4
Bamboo shoots	1 cup	41	1	4	8	3
Banana chips	1 oz.	147	10	1	17	2
Bananas	1 medium, 7"-8"	105	0	1	27	3
Barley	1 cup	651	4	23	135	32
Barley flour	1 cup	511	2	16	110	15
Barley, pearled, cooked	1 cup	193	1	4	44	6
Basil	5 leaves	1	0	0	0	0
Basil, dried	1 tsp	2	0	0	0	0
Bay leaf	1 tsp, crumbled	2	0	0	0	0
Beans, adzuki, cooked	1 cup	294	0	17	57	17
Beans, baked, canned, plain	1 cup	239	1	12	54	10
Beans, baked, canned, w/o salt	1 cup	266	1	12	52	13

Nutrition values for fat, protein (Prtn), carbohydrates (Cbs), and fiber (Fbr) are
listed in grams per serving. Serving sizes and values are approximate.

FOOD ITEM	SERVING SIZE	CAL	FAT	PRTN	CBS	FBR
B (CONT.)						
Beans, baked, canned, w/ beef	1 cup	322	9	17	45	10
Beans, black, cooked	1 cup	227	1	15	40	15
Beans, cranberry, cooked	1 cup	241	1	16	43	18
Beans, fava, canned	1 cup	182	1	14	31	10
Beans, french, cooked	1 cup	228	1	12	43	17
Beans, great northern, cooked	1 cup	209	1	15	37	12
Beans, kidney, cooked	1 cup	225	1	15	40	11
Beans, lima, cooked	1 cup	216	1	15	39	13
Beans, lima, canned	1 can	190	0	12	36	11
Beans, mung, cooked	1 cup	212	1	14	39	15
Beans, mungo, cooked	1 cup	189	1	14	33	12
Beans, navy, cooked	1 cup	255	1	15	47	19
Beans, pink, cooked	1 cup	252	1	15	47	9
Beans, pinto, cooked	1 cup	245	1	15	44	15
Beans, small white, cooked	1 cup	254	1	16	46	18
Beans, snap, green, cooked	1 cup	44	0	2	10	4
Beans, snap, yellow, cooked	1 cup	44	0	2	10	4
Beans, white, cooked	1 cup	249	1	17	45	11
Beans, yellow	1 cup	255	2	16	48	18
Beechnuts, dried	1 oz.	163	14	2	10	0
Beef, choice short rib, cooked	3 oz.	400	36	18	0	0
Beef bologna	1 slice	88	8	3	1	0
Beef jerky, chopped	1 piece	81	5	7	2	0
Beef sausage, precooked	1 link	134	12	6	1	0
Beef stew, canned	1 serving	218	13	12	16	4
Beef, tri-tip roast, roasted	3 oz.	174	9	22	0	0
Beef, brisket, lean and fat, roasted	3 oz.	328	27	20	0	0
Beef, brisket, lean, roasted	3 oz.	206	11	25	0	0
Beef, chuck, arm roast, lean & fat, braised	3 oz.	283	20	23	0	0
Beef, chuck, arm roast, lean, braised	3 oz.	179	7	28	0	0
Beef, chuck, top blade, raw	3 oz.	138	8	17	0	0
Beef, cured breakfast strips	3 slices	276	26	9	1	0
Beef, cured, corned, canned	3 oz.	213	13	23	0	0
Beef, cured, dried	1 serving	43	1	9	1	0
Beef, cured, luncheon meat	1 slice	31	1	5	0	0
Beef, flank, raw	1 oz.	47	2	6	0	0
Beef, ground patties, frozen	3 oz.	240	20	15	0	0
Beef, ground, 70% lean, raw	1 oz.	94	9	4	0	0
Beef, ground, 80% lean, raw	1 oz.	72	6	5	0	0
Beef, ground, 95% lean, raw	1 oz.	39	1	6	0	0
Beef, rib, large end, boneless, raw	1 oz.	94	8	5	0	0
Beef, rib, shortribs, boneless, raw	1 oz.	110	10	4	0	0
Beef, rib, whole, boneless, raw	1 oz.	91	8	5	0	0
Beef, rib-eye, small end, raw	1 oz.	78	6	5	0	0
Beef, round, bottom, raw	1 oz.	56	3	6	0	0
Beef, round, eye, raw	1 oz.	49	3	6	0	0
Beef, round, full cut, raw	1 oz.	55	3	6	0	0
Beef, round, tip, raw	1 oz.	56	4	6	0	0
Beef, round, top, raw	1 oz.	48	2	6	0	0
Beef, shank crosscuts, raw	1 oz.	50	3	6	0	0

Nutrition values for fat, protein (Prtn), carbohydrates (Cbs), and fiber (Fbr) are
listed in grams per serving. Serving sizes and values are approximate.

FOOD ITEM	SERVING SIZE	CAL	FAT	PRTN	CBS	FBR
B (CONT.)						
Beef, short loin, porterhouse, raw	1 oz.	73	6	5	0	0
Beef, short loin, t-bone, raw	1 oz.	66	5	5	0	0
Beef, short loin, top, raw	1 oz.	66	5	6	0	0
Beef, sirloin, tri-tip, raw	1 oz.	50	3	6	0	0
Beef, tenderloin, raw	1 oz.	70	5	6	0	0
Beef, top sirloin, raw	1 oz.	61	4	6	0	0
Beer, light	12 fl.oz.	110	12	5	7	0
Beer, nonalcoholic	12 fl.oz.	80	1	0	70	0
Beer, regular	12 fl.oz.	140	12	1	10	1
Beets	1 beet	35	0	2	8	4
Bratwurst, chicken	1 serving	148	9	16	0	0
Bratwurst, pork	1 serving	281	25	12	2	0
Bratwurst, veal	1 serving	286	27	12	0	0
Bread stuffing, dry mix, prepared	1/2 cup	178	9	3	22	3
Bread, banana	1 slice	196	6	3	33	1
Bread, corn	1 piece	188	6	4	29	1
Bread, cracked-wheat	1 slice	65	1	2	12	1
Bread, french	1 slice	70	1	3	15	1
Bread, garlic	1 slice	160	10	3	14	1
Bread, Irish soda	1 oz.	82	1	2	16	1
Bread, pita	2 oz.	150	1	3	30	0
Bread, pumpernickel	1 slice	75	1	3	15	2
Bread, raisin	1 slice	80	2	2	15	1
Bread, rice bran	1 oz.	69	1	3	12	1
Bread, sandwich slice	1 slice	70	1	2	13	1
Bread, sourdough	1 slice	100	1	2	20	1
Broad beans, cooked	1 cup	187	1	13	33	9
Brownies	1 brownie	220	13	1	27	1
Buckwheat	1 cup	583	6	23	122	17
Buckwheat flour	1 cup	402	4	15	85	12
Buckwheat groats, roasted, cooked	1 cup	155	1	6	34	5
Buffalo, raw	1 oz.	28	0	6	0	0
Burbot, raw	3 oz.	77	1	16	0	0
Burdock root	1 cup	85	0	2	21	4
Butter, whipped, w/ salt	1 tbsp	67	8	0	0	0
Butternuts, dried	1 oz.	174	16	7	3	1
C						
Cabbage, common	1 cup, shredded	17	1	1	4	2
Cabbage, pak choi	1 cup, shredded	9	0	1	2	1
Cabbage, pe-tsai	1 cup, shredded	12	0	1	3	1
Cake, angel food	1 slice	180	4	2	36	2
Cake, boston cream pie	1 slice	260	9	1	32	0
Cake, carrot	1 slice	310	16	1	39	0
Cake, cheesecake	1 slice	500	30	4	50	0
Cake, chocolate	1 slice	270	13	1	36	1
Cake, chocolate mousse	1 slice	250	10	1	35	1
Cake, devil's food	1 slice	270	13	2	35	0
Cake, pineapple upside-down	1 piece	367	14	4	58	1
Cake, pound	1 slice	320	16	2	38	0

Nutrition values for fat, protein (Prtn), carbohydrates (Cbs), and fiber (Fbr) are listed in grams per serving. Serving sizes and values are approximate.

FOOD ITEM	SERVING SIZE	CAL	FAT	PRTN	CBS	FBR
C (CONT.)						
Cake, sponge cake w/ cream, berries	1 slice	325	8	25	38	1
Cake, yellow	1 slice	260	11	2	36	1
Candy, butterscotch	5 pieces	120	3	0	20	0
Candy, caramels	1 piece	30	1	3	6	1
Candy, carob	1 bar	470	27	7	49	3
Candy, chocolate fudge	1 oz.	125	5	0	18	0
Candy, chocolate mints	1 mint	45	1	0	9	0
Candy, milk chocolate w/ almonds	2 oz.	216	14	4	21	3
Candy, chocolate-coated peanut butter bites	1 piece	45	3	1	4	0
Candy, chocolate-coated peanuts	12 peanuts	160	11	20	15	7
Candy, gumdrops	4 pieces	130	0	0	31	0
Candy, hard candy	1 piece	18	0	0	5	0
Candy, jelly beans	12 beans	100	0	0	24	0
Candy, licorice	1 piece	30	0	0	7	0
Candy, lollipop	1 lollipop	20	0	0	5	0
Candy, milk chocolate bar	2 oz.	235	13	3	26	2
Candy, mints	1 mint	30	0	0	7	0
Cantaloupe	1 cup, cubed	54	0	1	13	1
Cardoon	1 cup, shredded	36	0	1	9	3
Carrots	1 medium	65	0	1	15	4
Cashew butter, w/ salt	1 tbsp	94	8	3	4	0
Cashew nuts	1 oz.	157	12	5	9	1
Cassava	1 cup	330	1	3	78	4
Celeriac	1 cup	66	1	2	14	3
Chard, swiss	1 cup	7	0	1	1	1
Cheese, american	1 slice	110	9	5	1	0
Cheese, brick	1 oz.	100	8	31	0	0
Cheese, brie	1 oz.	95	8	50	1	0
Cheese, camembert	1 oz.	90	7	49	1	0
Cheese, cheddar	1 oz.	110	9	33	1	0
Cheese, colby jack	1 oz.	110	9	31	1	0
Cheese, cottage, 2%	1 cup	203	4	31	8	0
Cheese, edam	1 oz.	100	8	7	0	0
Cheese, feta	1 oz.	100	8	21	1	0
Cheese, goat	1 oz.	128	10	9	1	0
Cheese, goat, semisoft	1 oz.	103	9	6	1	0
Cheese, goat, soft	1 oz.	76	6	5	0	0
Cheese, gouda	1 oz.	100	8	7	1	0
Cheese, monterey jack	1 oz.	110	9	32	0	0
Cheese, moz.zarella	1 oz.	90	7	25	1	0
Cheese, parmesan, hard	1 oz.	110	7	10	1	0
Cheese, parmesan, shredded	1 tbsp	22	2	2	0	0
Cheese, provolone	1 oz.	100	8	34	1	0
Cheese, queso	2 tbsp	110	9	28	2	0
Cheese, ricotta	2 tbsp	50	4	28	1	0
Cheese, roquefort	1 oz.	105	9	6	1	0
Cheese, swiss	1 oz.	110	9	36	1	0
Cherries, sour	8 pieces	30	0	1	7	2
Cherries, sweet	8 pieces	30	0	2	7	2
Chewing gum	1 piece	25	0	0	5	0

Nutrition values for fat, protein (Prtn), carbohydrates (Cbs), and fiber (Fbr) are listed in grams per serving. Serving sizes and values are approximate.

FOOD ITEM	SERVING SIZE	CAL	FAT	PRTN	CBS	FBR
C (CONT.)						
Chicken, breast, w/ skin	1/2 breast	249	13	30	0	0
Chicken, breast, w/o skin	1/2 breast	130	2	27	0	0
Chicken, capons, boneless	1/2 capon	1459	74	184	0	0
Chicken, capons, giblets, cooked	1 cup	238	8	38	1	0
Chicken, cornish game hen, roasted	1/2 bird	336	24	29	0	0
Chicken, cornish game hen, meat only	1 bird	295	9	51	0	0
Chicken, dark meat, w/o skin	1 cup diced	287	14	38	0	0
Chicken, drumstick, w/ skin	1 drumstick	118	6	14	0	0
Chicken, drumstick, w/o skin	1 drumstick	74	2	13	0	0
Chicken, leg, w/ skin	1 leg	312	20	30	0	0
Chicken, leg, w/o skin	1 leg	156	5	26	0	0
Chicken, light meat, w/o skin	1 cup diced	214	6	38	0	0
Chicken, thigh, w/ skin	1 thigh	198	14	16	0	0
Chicken, thigh, w/o skin	1 thigh	82	3	14	0	0
Chicken, wing, w/ skin	1 wing	109	8	9	0	0
Chicken, wing, w/o skin	1 wing	37	1	6	0	0
Chickpeas, cooked	1 cup	269	4	15	45	13
Chicory greens	1 cup, chopped	41	1	3	9	7
Chicory roots	1/2 cup	33	0	1	8	0
Chicory, witloof	1/2 cup	8	0	0	2	1
Chili con carne w/ beans	1 cup	298	13	18	28	10
Chili powder	1 tsp	8	0	0	1	1
Chili w/ beans, canned	1 cup	287	14	15	31	11
Chili w/o beans, canned	1 cup	194	7	17	18	3
Chinese chestnuts	1 oz.	64	0	1	14	0
Chives	1 tbsp, chopped	1	0	0	0	0
Chocolate chip crisped rice bar	1 bar	115	4	1	21	1
Chocolate chips	1/4 cup	210	12	3	24	1
Chocolate milkshake, ready-to-drink	8 fl.oz.	181	5	8	26	1
Chocolate, semi sweet bars, baking	1 oz.	160	8	3	20	1
Chocolate, unsweetened baking squares	1 square	144	15	4	9	5
Chorizo, pork and beef	1 link	273	23	15	1	0
Chow mein noodles	1 cup	237	14	4	26	2
Cinnamon, ground	1 tsp	6	0	0	2	1
Cisco	3 oz.	83	2	16	0	0
Citrus fruit drink, from concentrate	8 fl.oz.	124	0	1	30	1
Clam, mixed species, raw	1 large	15	0	3	1	0
Cloves, ground	1 tsp	7	0	0	1	1
Cocktail mix, nonalcoholic	1 fl.oz.	103	0	0	26	0
Cocoa mix, powder	1 serving	113	1	2	24	1
Cocoa mix, powder, unsweetened	1 tbsp	12	1	1	3	2
Coconut meat	1 cup, shredded	283	27	3	12	7
Coconut milk	1 cup	552	57	6	13	5
Coffee, brewed, decaf	1 cup	0	0	0	0	0
Coffee, brewed, regular	1 cup	2	0	0	0	0
Coffee, café au lait	8 fl.oz.	65	3	1	6	0
Coffee, cappuccino	8 fl.oz.	70	4	1	6	0
Coffee, espresso	1 shot	4	0	0	1	0
Coffee, instant, decaf	1 tsp	0	0	0	0	0
Coffee, instant, regular	1 tsp, dry	2	0	0	0	0

Nutrition values for fat, protein (Prtn), carbohydrates (Cbs), and fiber (Fbr) are listed in grams per serving. Serving sizes and values are approximate.

FOOD ITEM	SERVING SIZE	CAL	FAT	PRTN	CBS	FBR
C (CONT.)						
Coffee, latte	8 fl.oz.	100	5	0	8	0
Coffee, mocha	8 fl.oz.	180	12	1	16	0
Coffeecake	3 oz.	230	7	4	38	4
Coleslaw	1/2 cup	41	2	1	7	1
Collards	1 cup, chopped	11	0	1	2	1
Conch, baked or broiled	1 cup, sliced	165	2	33	2	0
Cookies, animal crackers	1 cookie	22	1	0	4	0
Cookies, brownies	4 oz.	430	25	1	52	1
Cookies, butter	1 cookie	23	1	0	3	0
Cookies, chocolate chip, deli fresh baked	1 cookie	275	15	0	38	1
Cookies, chocolate chip, commercial	1 cookie	130	7	1	17	1
Cookies, chocolate chip, refrigerated dough	1 portion	128	6	1	18	0
Cookies, chocolate wafers	1 wafer	26	1	0	4	0
Cookies, fig bars	1 cookie	150	3	2	31	2
Cookies, fudge	1 cookie	73	1	1	16	1
Cookies, gingersnap	1 cookie	29	1	0	5	0
Cookies, graham, plain or honey	2 1/2" square	30	1	1	5	0
Cookies, marshmallow w/ chocolate coating	1 cookie	118	5	1	19	1
Cookies, molasses	1 cookie	138	4	2	24	0
Cookies, oatmeal	1 cookie	238	9	3	38	2
Cookies, oatmeal w/ raisins	1 cookie	238	9	3	38	2
Cookies, oatmeal, commercial, iced	1 cookie	123	5	1	18	1
Cookies, oatmeal, refrigerated dough	1 portion	68	3	1	10	0
Cookies, peanut butter sandwich	1 cookie	67	3	1	9	0
Cookies, peanut butter, refrigerated dough	1 portion	73	4	1	8	0
Cookies, sugar	1 cookie	66	3	1	8	0
Cookies, sugar wafers w/ cream filling	1 wafer	46	2	0	6	0
Cookies, sugar, refrigerated dough	1 portion	113	5	1	15	0
Cookies, vanilla wafers	1 wafer	28	1	0	4	0
Coriander leaves	9 sprigs	5	0	0	1	1
Corn flour, yellow	1 cup	416	4	11	87	0
Corn, sweet, white	1 ear	77	1	3	17	2
Corn, sweet, yellow	1 ear	77	1	3	17	2
Corn, sweet, white, cream style	1 cup	184	1	5	46	3
Corn, sweet, yellow, cream style	1 cup	184	1	5	46	3
Cornnuts	1 oz.	126	4	2	20	2
Cornstarch	1 cup	488	0	0	117	1
Couscous, cooked	1 cup	176	0	6	37	0
Cowpeas (black-eyed peas), cooked	1 cup	160	1	5	34	8
Cowpeas, catjang, cooked	1 cup	200	1	14	35	6
Cowpeas, leafy tips	1 cup, chopped	10	0	2	2	0
Crab, alaska king, raw	1 leg	144	1	32	0	0
Crab, blue, canned	1 cup	134	2	28	0	0
Crab, dungeness, cooked	1 crab	140	2	28	1	0
Crabapples	1 cup, sliced	84	0	0	22	0
Crackers w/ cheese filling	6 crackers	191	10	4	23	1
Crackers w/ peanut butter filling	6 cracker	193	10	5	22	1
Crackers, cheese, regular	6 crackers	312	16	6	36	2
Crackers, graham	1 cracker	30	1	6	5	2
Crackers, matzo, plain	1 matzo	112	0	3	24	1

Nutrition values for fat, protein (Prtn), carbohydrates (Cbs), and fiber (Fbr) are
listed in grams per serving. Serving sizes and values are approximate.

FOOD ITEM	SERVING SIZE	CAL	FAT	PRTN	CBS	FBR
C (CONT.)						
Crackers, matzo, whole-wheat	1 matzo	100	0	4	22	3
Crackers, melba toast	1 cup	129	1	4	25	2
Crackers, milk	1 cracker	50	2	1	8	0
Crackers, regular	1 cup, bite size	311	16	5	38	1
Crackers, rusk toast	1 rusk	41	1	1	7	0
Crackers, rye	1 cracker	37	0	1	9	3
Crackers, saltines	1 cracker	20	0	1	4	0
Crackers, soda	1 cracker	60	2	6	10	2
Crackers, wheat	1 cracker	9	0	0	1	0
Crackers, wheat, sandwich w/ peanut butter	1 cracker	35	2	1	4	0
Crackers, whole-wheat	1 cracker	18	1	0	3	0
Cranberries	1 cup, whole	44	0	0	12	4
Cranberry juice cocktail	1 cup	144	0	0	36	0
Cranberry-apple juice	1 cup	174	0	0	44	0
Cranberry-grape juice	1 cup	137	0	1	34	0
Crayfish, wild, raw	8 crayfish	21	0	4	0	0
Cream cheese	1 tbsp	51	5	1	0	0
Cream of tartar	1 tsp	8	0	0	2	0
Cream, half & half	1 tbsp	20	2	0	1	0
Cream, heavy whipping	1 cup, fluid	821	88	5	7	0
Crepes	1 crepe	120	6	2	14	1
Croissants, apple	1 croissant	145	5	4	21	1
Croissants, butter	1 croissant	115	6	2	13	1
Croissants, cheese	1 croissant	174	9	4	20	1
Croutons, plain	1 cup	122	2	4	22	2
Croutons, seasoned	1 cup	186	7	4	25	2
Cucumber	1 cucumber	45	0	2	11	2
Cucumber, peeled	1 cup, sliced	14	0	1	3	1
Cumin seed	1 tsp	8	1	0	1	0
Currants, black	1 cup	71	1	2	17	0
Currants, red & white	1 cup	63	0	2	16	5
Curry powder	1 tsp	7	0	0	1	1
D						
Dandelion greens	1 cup, chopped	25	0	2	5	2
Danish pastry, cheese, 4 1/4" diameter	1 pastry	266	16	6	26	1
Danish pastry, cinnamon, 4 1/4" diameter	1 pastry	262	15	5	29	1
Danish pastry, fruit, 4 1/4" diameter	1 pastry	263	13	4	34	1
Danish pastry, nut, 4 1/4" diameter	1 pastry	280	16	5	30	1
Danish pastry, raspberry, 4 1/4" diameter	1 pastry	263	13	4	34	1
Deer, ground, raw	1 oz.	45	2	6	0	0
Deer, raw	1 oz.	34	1	7	0	0
Doughnuts, chocolate coated or frosted	1 doughnut	133	9	1	13	1
Doughnuts, chocolate, sugared or glazed	1 doughnut	250	12	3	34	1
Doughnuts, french crullers	1 cruller	169	8	1	24	1
Doughnuts, plain	1 doughnut, stick	219	12	3	26	1
Doughnuts, wheat, sugared or glazed	1 doughnut	101	5	2	12	1
Duck liver, raw	1 liver	60	2	8	2	0
Duck, meat only, roasted	1/2 duck	444	25	52	0	0
Duck, white pekin, breast w/skin, roasted	1/2 breast	242	13	29	0	0

Nutrition values for fat, protein (Prtn), carbohydrates (Cbs), and fiber (Fbr) are listed in grams per serving. Serving sizes and values are approximate.

FOOD ITEM	SERVING SIZE	CAL	FAT	PRTN	CBS	FBR
D (CONT.)						
Duck, skinless, raw	1/2 duck	400	18	55	0	0
Durian	1 cup, chopped	357	13	4	66	9
E						
Eclairs w/ chocolate glaze	1 éclair	293	18	7	27	1
Eel, mixed species, raw	3 oz.	156	10	16	0	0
Egg noodles, cooked	1 cup	213	2	8	40	2
Egg substitute, liquid	1 tbsp	13	1	2	0	0
Egg white, fried	1 large	92	7	6	0	0
Egg white, raw	1 large	17	0	4	0	0
Egg yolk, raw	1 large	53	4	3	1	0
Egg, hard-boiled	1 cup, chopped	211	14	17	2	0
Egg, omelette	1 large	93	7	7	0	0
Egg, poached	1 large	74	5	6	0	0
Egg, raw	1 large	85	5.8	7	0	0
Egg, scrambled	1 cup	365	27	24	5	0
Eggnog	8 fl.oz.	343	19	10	34	0
Eggplant	1 eggplant	110	10	5	26	16
Elderberries	1 cup	106	1	1	27	10
Elk, ground, raw	1 oz.	49	3	6	0	0
Elk, raw	1 oz.	31	0	7	0	0
Endive	1 head	87	1	6	17	16
English muffins, plain	1 muffin	134	1	4	26	2
English muffins, cinnamon-raisin	1 muffin	139	2	4	49	2
English muffins, wheat	1 muffin	127	1	5	26	3
English muffins, whole-wheat	1 muffin	134	1	6	27	4
English muffins, whole-wheat/multigrain	1 muffin	155	1	6	31	2
European chestnuts, peeled	1 oz.	56	0	1	13	0
European chestnuts, unpeeled	1 oz.	60	1	1	13	2
F						
Farina, cooked	1 cup.	471	0	3	24	1
Fast food, biscuit w/ egg	1 biscuit	373	22	12	32	1
Fast food, biscuit w/ egg & bacon	1 biscuit	458	31	17	29	1
Fast food, biscuit w/ egg, bacon & cheese	1 biscuit	477	31	16	33	0
Fast food, biscuit w/ sausage	1 biscuit	485	32	12	40	1
Fast food, caramel sundae	1 sundae	304	9	7	49	0
Fast food, cheeseburger, large, double patty	1 sandwich	704	44	38	40	1
Fast food, cheeseburger, large, single patty	1 sandwich	563	33	28	38	1
Fast food, corndog	1 corndog	460	19	17	56	1
Fast food, croissant w/ egg, cheese	1 croissant	368	25	13	24	1
Fast food, croissant w/ egg, cheese, bacon	1 croissant	413	28	16	24	1
Fast food, croissant w/ egg, cheese, sausage	1 croissant	523	38	20	25	1
Fast food, Danish pastry, cheese	1 pastry	353	25	6	29	2
Fast food, Danish pastry, cinnamon	1 pastry	349	17	5	47	2
Fast food, Danish pastry, fruit	1 pastry	335	16	5	45	2
Fast food, fish sandwich w/ tartar sauce	1 sandwich	431	23	17	41	1
Fast food, french toast sticks	5 pieces	513	29	8	58	3
Fast food, fried chicken, boneless	6 pieces	285	18	15	16	1
Fast food, hamburger, large, double patty	1 sandwich	540	27	34	40	2

Nutrition values for fat, protein (Prtn), carbohydrates (Cbs), and fiber (Fbr) are
listed in grams per serving. Serving sizes and values are approximate.

FOOD ITEM	SERVING SIZE	CAL	FAT	PRTN	CBS	FBR
F (CONT.)						
Fast food, hamburger, large, single patty	1 sandwich	425	21	23	37	2
Fast food, hot fudge sundae	1 sundae	284	9	6	48	0
Fast food, hot dog w/ chili	1 hot dog	296	13	14	31	1
Fast food, hot dog, plain	1 hot dog	242	15	10	18	1
Fast food, McDonald's Big Mac® w/ cheese	1 serving	560	30	25	46	3
Fast food, McDonald's Big Mac® w/o cheese	1 serving	495	25	23	43	3
Fast food, McDonald's cheeseburger	1 serving	310	12	15	35	1
Fast food, McDonald's Chicken McGrill®	1 serving	400	16	27	38	3
Fast food, McDonald's Crispy Chicken	1 serving	500	23	24	50	3
Fast food, McDonald's Filet-o-Fish®	1 serving	400	18	14	42	1
Fast food, McDonald's french fries	1 medium	350	11	4	47	5
Fast food, McDonald's hamburger	1 serving	260	9	13	33	1
Fast food, McDonald's 1/4 Pounder®,cheese	1 serving	510	25	29	43	3
Fast food, McDonald's 1/4 Pounder®	1 serving	420	18	24	40	3
Fast food, onion rings, 8-9 rings	1 portion	276	16	4	31	3
Fast food, strawberry sundae	1 sundae	268	8	6	45	0
Fast food, submarine sandwich w/ cold cuts	1 submarine 6"	456	19	22	51	4
Fast food, submarine sandwich w/ roast beef	1 submarine 6"	410	13	29	44	4
Fast food, submarine sandwich w/ tuna	1 submarine 6"	584	28	30	55	4
Fast food, vanilla soft-serve w/ cone	1 cone	164	6	4	24	0
Fennel bulb	1 cup, sliced	27	0	1	6	3
Fennel seed	1 tbsp	20	1	1	3	2
Fenugreek seed	1 tbsp	36	1	3	7	3
Figs	1 medium	37	0	0	10	2
Figs, dried	1 fig	21	0	0	5	1
Fireweed leaves	1 cup, chopped	24	1	1	4	2
Fish oil, cod liver	1 tbsp	123	14	0	0	0
Fish oil, herring	1 tbsp	123	14	0	0	0
Fish oil, menhaden	1 tbsp	123	14	0	0	0
Fish oil, salmon	1 tbsp	123	14	0	0	0
Fish oil, sardine	1 tbsp	123	14	0	0	0
Fish, bluefin tuna, raw	3 oz.	122	4	20	0	0
Fish, bluefish, raw	3 oz.	105	4	17	0	0
Fish, butterfish, raw	3 oz.	124	7	15	0	0
Fish, carp, raw	3 oz.	108	5	15	0	0
Fish, catfish, raw	3 oz.	81	2	14	0	0
Fish, cod, atlantic, raw	3 oz.	70	1	15	0	0
Fish, croaker, atlantic, raw	3 oz.	88	3	15	0	0
Fish, flatfish, raw	3 oz.	77	1	16	0	0
Fish, gefilte fish	1 piece	35	1	4	3	0
Fish, grouper, mixed species, raw	3 oz.	78	1	17	0	0
Fish, haddock, raw	3 oz.	74	1	16	0	0
Fish, halibut, raw	3 oz.	94	2	18	0	0
Fish, herring, atlantic, raw	3 oz.	134	8	15	0	0
Fish, herring, pacific, raw	3 oz.	166	12	14	0	0
Fish, mackerel, atlantic, raw	3 oz.	174	12	16	0	0
Fish, mackerel, king, raw	3 oz.	89	2	17	0	0
Fish, mackerel, pacific, raw	3 oz.	134	7	17	0	0
Fish, mackerel, spanish, raw	3 oz.	118	5	16	0	0
Fish, milkfish, raw	3 oz.	126	6	18	0	0

Nutrition values for fat, protein (Prtn), carbohydrates (Cbs), and fiber (Fbr) are listed in grams per serving. Serving sizes and values are approximate.

FOOD ITEM	SERVING SIZE	CAL	FAT	PRTN	CBS	FBR
F (CONT.)						
Fish, monkfish, raw	3 oz.	65	1	12	0	0
Fish, ocean perch, atlantic, raw	3 oz.	80	1	16	0	0
Fish, perch, mixed species, raw	3 oz.	77	1	17	0	0
Fish, pike, northern, raw	3 oz.	75	1	16	0	0
Fish, pollock, atlantic, raw	3 oz.	78	1	17	0	0
Fish, pout, ocean, raw	3 oz.	67	1	14	0	0
Fish, rainbow smelt, raw	3 oz.	82	2	15	0	0
Fish, rockfish, pacific, raw	3 oz.	80	1	16	0	0
Fish, roe, mixed species, raw	1 tbsp	20	10	3	0	0
Fish, sablefish, raw	3 oz.	166	13	11	0	0
Fish, salmon, atlantic, farmed, raw	3 oz.	156	9	17	0	0
Fish, salmon, atlantic, wild, raw	3 oz.	121	5	17	0	0
Fish, salmon, chinook, raw	3 oz.	152	9	17	0	0
Fish, salmon, pink, raw	3 oz.	99	3	17	0	0
Fish, sea bass, mixed species, raw	3 oz.	82	2	16	0	0
Fish, seatrout, mixed species, raw	3 oz.	88	3	14	0	0
Fish, shad, raw	3 oz.	167	12	14	0	0
Fish, skipjack tuna, raw	3 oz.	88	1	19	0	0
Fish, snapper, mixed species, raw	3 oz.	85	1	17	0	0
Fish, striped bass, raw	3 oz.	82	2	15	0	0
Fish, striped mullet	3 oz.	99	3	16	0	0
Fish, sturgeon, mixed species, raw	3 oz.	89	3	14	0	0
Fish, swordfish, raw	3 oz.	103	3	17	0	0
Fish, trout, mixed species, raw	3 oz.	126	6	18	0	0
Fish, white sucker, raw	3 oz.	78	2	14	0	0
Fish, whitefish, raw	3 oz.	114	5	16	0	0
Fish, wolffish, atlantic, raw	3 oz.	82	2	15	0	0
Fish, yellowfin tuna, raw	3 oz.	93	1	20	0	0
Fish, yellowtail, mixed species, raw	3 oz.	124	5	20	0	0
Flan, caramel custard	5 1/2 oz.	303	12	4	43	0
Flaxseed	1 tbsp	59	4	2	4	3
Flaxseed oil	1 tbsp	120	14	0	0	0
Frankfurter	1 serving	151	13	5	2	0
Frankfurter, beef	1 frankfurter	188	17	6	2	0
Frankfurter, beef & pork	1 frankfurter	174	16	7	1	1
Frankfurter, chicken	1 frankfurter	116	9	6	3	0
Frankfurter, meat	1 frankfurter	151	13	5	2	0
Frankfurter, meatless	1 frankfurter	163	10	14	5	3
Frankfurter, pork	1 frankfurter	204	18	10	0	0
Frankfurter, turkey	1 frankfurter	102	8	6	1	0
French fries, frozen, unprepared, 18 fries	1 serving	170	7	3	28	3
French toast, frozen, ready-to-heat	1 piece	126	4	4	19	1
Frosting, creamy chocolate	2 tbsp	164	7	1	26	0
Frosting, creamy vanilla	2 tbsp	160	6	0	26	0
Frozen yogurt, chocolate, soft-serve	1/2 cup	115	4	3	18	2
Frozen yogurt, vanilla, soft-serve	1/2 cup	117	4	3	17	0
Fruit cocktail, canned	1 cup	229	0	1	60	3
Fruit punch, prepared from concentrate	8 fl.oz.	124	1	0	30	0
Fruit salad, canned in syrup	1 cup	186	0	1	49	3
Fruit salad, canned in water	1 cup	74	0	1	19	3

Nutrition values for fat, protein (Prtn), carbohydrates (Cbs), and fiber (Fbr) are listed in grams per serving. Serving sizes and values are approximate.

NUTRITION FACTS

FOOD ITEM	SERVING SIZE	CAL	FAT	PRTN	CBS	FBR
G						
Garden cress, raw	1 cup	16	0	1	3	1
Garlic	1 clove	4	0	0	1	0
Garlic powder	1 tsp	9	0	1	2	0
Gelatin dessert mix, prepared w/ water	1/2 cup	84	0	2	19	0
Gin, 80 Proof	1 fl.oz.	73	0	0	0	0
Ginger root	1 tsp	2	0	0	0	0
Ginger, ground	1 tsp	6	0	0	1	0
Ginkgo nuts	1 oz.	52	1	1	11	0
Ginkgo nuts, dried	1 oz.	99	1	3	21	0
Goose liver, raw	1 liver	125	4	15	6	0
Goose, meat & skin, roasted	cup chopped	427	31	35	0	0
Goose, meat only, roasted	cup chopped	340	18	41	0	0
Gourd, white-flowered	1 gourd	108	0	5	26	0
Granola bars, hard, plain	1 bar	134	6	3	18	2
Granola bars, soft, plain	1 bar	126	5	2	19	1
Grape juice	8 fl.oz.	160	0	0	40	0
Grapefruit	1/2 fruit	50	0	1	12	3
Grapefruit juice, sweetened	8 fl.oz.	125	0	0	33	0
Grapefruit juice, unsweetened	8 fl.oz.	91	0	1	22	0
Grapes, canned, heavy syrup	1 cup	187	0	1	50	2
Grapes, red or green	1 cup	106	0	1	28	1
Gravy, mushroom, canned	1 can	149	8	4	16	1
Gravy, au jus, canned	1 can	48	1	4	8	0
Gravy, beef, canned	1 can	154	7	11	14	1
Gravy, chicken, canned	1 can	235	17	6	16	1
Gravy, turkey, canned	1 can	152	6	8	15	1
Guacamole dip	2 tbsp	50	4	12	4	0
Guavas	1 fruit	37	1	1	8	3
H						
Ham, chopped	1 slice	50	3	5	1	0
Ham, minced	1 slice	55	4	3	0	0
Ham, sliced	1 slice	46	2	5	1	0
Hazlenuts, dry roasted	1 oz.	183	18	4	5	3
Hazlenuts, blanched	1 oz.	178	17	4	5	3
Hominy, canned, white	1 cup	119	2	2	24	4
Hominy, canned, yellow	1 cup	115	1	2	23	4
Honey	1 tbsp	64	0	0	17	0
Honeydew melons	1 cup, diced	61	0	1	16	1
Horseradish	1 tsp	2	0	0	1	0
Hot chocolate	8 fl.oz.	200	10	9	25	3
Hummus	1 tbsp	23	1	1	2	1
Hush puppies	1 hush puppy	74	3	2	10	1
I						
Ice cream cone, rolled or sugar type	1 cone	40	0	1	8	0
Ice cream cone, wafer or cake type	1 cone	17	0	0	3	0
Ice cream, chocolate	1/2 cup	143	7	3	19	1
Ice cream, strawberry	1/2 cup	127	6	2	18	1
Ice cream, vanilla	1/2 cup	144	8	3	17	1

Nutrition values for fat, protein (Prtn), carbohydrates (Cbs), and fiber (Fbr) are listed in grams per serving. Serving sizes and values are approximate.

FOOD ITEM	SERVING SIZE	CAL	FAT	PRTN	CBS	FBR
I (CONT.)						
Iced tea, presweetened	8 fl.oz.	100	0	0	25	0
Iced tea, unsweetened	8 fl.oz.	2	0	0	0	0
Italian seasoning	1 tsp	4	0	0	1	0
J						
Jams and preserves	1 tbsp	56	0	0	14	0
Japanese chestnuts	1 oz.	44	0	1	10	0
Japanese soba noodles, cooked	1 cup	113	0	6	24	2
Japanese ramen noodles, packaged, dry	1 serving	195	7	4	28	1
Jellies	1 tbsp	55	0	0	14	0
K						
Kale	1 cup, chopped	34	1	2	7	1
Kiwifruit	1 medium	45	0	2	11	5
Kumquats	1 fruit	13	0	0	3	1
L						
Lamb, cubed, raw	1 oz.	38	2	6	0	0
Lamb, foreshank, raw	1 oz.	57	4	5	0	0
Lamb, ground, raw	1 oz.	80	7	5	0	0
Lamb, leg, shank half, raw	1 oz.	52	3	5	0	0
Lamb, leg, sirloin half, raw	1 oz.	74	6	5	0	0
Lamb, leg, whole, choice, raw	1 oz.	65	5	5	0	0
Lamb, loin, choice, raw	1 oz.	79	6	5	0	0
Lamb, rib, choice, raw	1 oz.	97	9	4	0	0
Lamb, shoulder, arm, raw	1 oz.	69	5	5	0	0
Lamb, shoulder, blade, raw	1 oz.	69	5	5	0	0
Lamb, shoulder, whole, raw	1 oz.	69	5	5	0	0
Lard	1 tbsp	115	13	0	0	0
Leeks	1 leek	54	0	1	13	2
Lemon juice	1 cup	61	0	1	21	1
Lemon juice, canned or bottled	1 tbsp	3	0	0	1	0
Lemon pepper seasoning	1 tsp	7	0	0	1	0
Lemonade powder	1 scoop	102	0	0	27	0
Lemonade, pink concentrate, prepared	8 fl.oz.	99	0	0	26	0
Lemonade, white concentrate, prepared	8 fl.oz.	131	0	0	34	0
Lemons w/ peel	1 fruit	22	0	1	12	5
Lentils, cooked	1 cup	230	1	18	40	16
Lentils, sprouted, raw	1 cup	82	0	7	17	0
Lettuce, green leaf	1 cup, shredded	5	0	1	1	1
Lettuce, iceberg	1 cup, shredded	10	0	1	2	1
Lettuce, red leaf	1 cup, shredded	3	0	0	0	0
Lettuce, romaine	1 cup, shredded	8	0	1	2	1
Lime juice	1 cup	62	0	1	21	1
Limes	1 fruit	20	0	1	7	2
Liverwurst, pork	1 slice	59	5	3	0	0
Lobster, northern, raw	1 lobster	135	1	28	1	0
Luncheon meat, beef, loaved	1 oz.	87	7	4	1	0
Luncheon meat, beef, thin sliced	1 oz.	50	1	8	2	0
Luncheon meat, meatless slices	1 slice	26	2	3	1	0

Nutrition values for fat, protein (Prtn), carbohydrates (Cbs), and fiber (Fbr) are
listed in grams per serving. Serving sizes and values are approximate.

FOOD ITEM	SERVING SIZE	CAL	FAT	PRTN	CBS	FBR
L (CONT.)						
Luncheon meat, pork & chicken, minced	1 oz.	56	4	4	0	0
Luncheon meat, pork & ham, minced	1 oz.	88	75	4	1	0
Luncheon meat, pork or beef	1 oz.	99	9	4	1	0
Luncheon meat, pork, canned	1 oz.	95	9	4	1	0
Luncheon meat, pork, ham & chicken, minced	1 oz.	87	8	4	1	0
Luncheon sausage, pork & beef	1 oz.	74	6	4	0	0
M						
Macadamia nuts	1 oz. (10-12 nuts)	203	22	2	4	2
Macaroni and cheese, commercial, prepared	1 cup	259	3	11	48	2
Macaroni, cooked	1 cup	197	1	7	40	2
Malt drink mix, dry	3 heaping tsp	87	2	2	16	0
Malt beverage	8 fl.oz.	144	0	1	32	0
Mangos	1 fruit	135	1	1	35	4
Maraschino cherries	1 cherry	8	0	0	2	0
Margarine, fat free spread	1 tbsp	6	0	0	1	0
Margarine, stick	1 tbsp	100	11	0	0	0
Margarine, stick, unsalted	1 tbsp	102	11	0	0	0
Margarine, tub	1 tbsp	102	11	0	0	0
Martini	1 fl.oz.	69	0	0	1	0
Mayonnaise	1 tbsp	100	11	0	0	0
Milk, 1% low fat	1 cup	102	2	8	12	0
Milk, 2% low fat	1 cup	138	5	10	14	0
Milk, buttermilk, cultured, reduced fat	1 cup	137	5	10	13	0
Milk, chocolate	1 cup	208	9	8	26	2
Milk, dry, nonfat, instant	1/3 cup dry	82	0	8	12	0
Milk, evaporated	1/2 cup	169	10	9	13	0
Milk, skim or nonfat	1 cup	83	0	8	12	0
Milk, canned, sweetened condensed	1 cup	982	27	24	167	0
Milk, whole	1 cup	146	8	8	11	0
Milkshake, dry mix, vanilla	1 envelope packet	69	1	5	11	0
Millet	1 cup	756	8	22	146	17
Miso soup	1 cup	547	17	32	73	15
Mixed nuts	1 cup	814	71	24	35	12
Molasses	1 tablespoon	58	0	0	15	0
Muffins, apple bran	1 muffin	300	3	1	61	1
Muffins, banana nut	1 muffin	480	24	3	60	2
Muffins, blueberry	1 muffin	313	7	6	54	3
Muffins, chocolate chip	1 muffin	510	24	2	69	4
Muffins, corn	1 muffin	345	10	7	58	4
Muffins, oat bran	1 muffin	305	8	8	55	5
Muffins, plain	1 muffin	242	9	4	36	2
Mushrooms	1 cup, pieces	15	0	2	2	1
Mushrooms, enoki	1 large	2	0	0	0	0
Mushrooms, oyster	1 large	55	1	6	9	4
Mushrooms, portobello	1 large	0	0	0	0	0
Mushrooms, shiitake	1 mushroom	11	0	0	3	0
Mussels, blue, raw	1 cup	129	3	18	6	0
Mustard greens	1 cup, chopped	15	0	2	3	2
Mustard seed, yellow	1 tbsp	53	3	3	4	2

Nutrition values for fat, protein (Prtn), carbohydrates (Cbs), and fiber (Fbr) are listed in grams per serving. Serving sizes and values are approximate.

FOOD ITEM	SERVING SIZE	CAL	FAT	PRTN	CBS	FBR
M (CONT.)						
Mustard spinach	1 cup, chopped	33	1	3	6	4
Mustard, prepared, yellow	1 tsp	3	0	0	0	0
N						
Natto (fermented soybeans)	1 cup	371	19	31	25	10
Nectarines	1 fruit	60	0	1	14	2
New Zealand spinach	1 cup, chopped	8	0	1	1	0
Nutmeg, ground	1 tsp	12	1	0	1	1
O						
Oat bran	1 cup	231	7	16	62	15
Oatmeal, instant, prepared w/ water	1 cup	129	2	5	22	4
Oil, canola	1 tbsp	124	14	0	0	0
Oil, canola & soybean	1 tbsp	119	14	0	0	0
Oil, coconut	1 tbsp	120	14	0	0	0
Oil, corn, peanut & olive	1 tbsp	120	14	0	0	0
Oil, olive	1 tbsp	119	14	0	0	0
Oil, peanut	1 tbsp	119	14	0	0	0
Oil, sesame	1 tbsp	120	14	0	0	0
Oil, soy	1 tbsp	120	14	0	0	0
Oil, vegetable, almond	1 tbsp	120	14	0	0	0
Oil, vegetable, cocoa butter	1 tbsp	120	14	0	0	0
Oil, vegetable, coconut	1 tbsp	117	14	0	0	0
Oil, vegetable, grapeseed	1 tbsp	120	14	0	0	0
Oil, vegetable, hazelnut	1 tbsp	120	14	0	0	0
Oil, vegetable, nutmeg butter	1 tbsp	120	14	0	0	0
Oil, vegetable, palm	1 tbsp	120	14	0	0	0
Oil, vegetable, poppyseed	1 tbsp	120	14	0	0	0
Oil, vegetable, rice bran	1 tbsp	120	14	0	0	0
Oil, vegetable, sheanut	1 tbsp	120	14	0	0	0
Oil, vegetable, tomatoseed	1 tbsp	120	14	0	0	0
Oil, vegetable, walnut	1 tbsp	120	14	0	0	0
Okra	1 cup	31	0	2	7	3
Onion powder	1 tsp	8	0	0	2	0
Onions	1 cup, chopped	67	0	2	16	2
Onions, sweet	1 onion	106	0	3	25	3
Orange juice	8 fl.oz.	109	1	2	25	1
Orange marmalade	1 tbsp	49	0	0	13	0
Oranges	1 large	86	0	2	22	4
Oregano, dried	1 tsp, ground	6	0	0	1	1
Oyster, eastern, raw	3 oz.	50	1	4	5	0
Oyster, pacific, raw	3 oz.	69	2	8	4	0
P						
Pancakes, blueberry	1 pancake	84	4	2	11	0
Pancakes, buttermilk	1 pancake	86	4	3	11	0
Pancakes, plain, dry mix	1 pancake	74	1	2	14	1
Papayas	1 cup, cubed	55	0	1	14	3
Paprika	1 tsp	6	0	0	1	1
Parsley	1 cup	22	1	2	4	2

Nutrition values for fat, protein (Prtn), carbohydrates (Cbs), and fiber (Fbr) are listed in grams per serving. Serving sizes and values are approximate.

FOOD ITEM	SERVING SIZE	CAL	FAT	PRTN	CBS	FBR
P (CONT.)						
Parsley, dried	1 tsp	1	0	0	0	0
Parsnips	1 cup, sliced	100	0	2	24	7
Passion fruit	1 fruit	17	0	0	4	2
Pasta, corn, cooked	1 cup	176	1	4	39	7
Pasta, plain, cooked	1 cup	197	1	7	40	2
Pasta, spinach, cooked	1 cup	195	1	8	38	2
Pastrami, turkey	1 oz.	40	2	5	1	0
Pate de foie gras	1 tbsp	60	6	2	1	0
Pate, chicken liver, canned	1 tbsp	26	2	2	1	0
Pate, goose liver, canned	1 tbsp	60	6	2	1	0
Peaches	1 large	61	0	1	15	2
Peaches, canned	1 cup, halved	59	0	1	15	3
Peanut butter, chunky	2 tbsp	188	16	8	7	3
Peanut butter, smooth	2 tbsp	188	16	8	6	2
Peanuts, dry roasted w/ salt	1 oz.	166	14	7	6	2
Peanuts, raw	1 oz.	161	14	7	5	2
Pears	1 pear	121	0	1	32	7
Pears, asian	1 pear	116	1	1	29	10
Pears, canned	1 cup	71	0	1	19	4
Peas, green, fresh, cooked	1 cup	134	0	9	25	9
Peas, green, frozen, cooked	1 cup	125	0	8	23	9
Peas, split, cooked	1 cup	231	1	16	41	16
Pecans	1 oz. (20 halves)	196	20	3	40	3
Pepper, black	1 tsp	5	0	0	1	1
Pepper, red or cayenne	1 tsp	6	0	0	1	1
Pepperoni	15 slices	135	12	6	1	0
Peppers, chili, green	1 cup	29	0	1	6	2
Peppers, chili, red	1 pepper	18	0	1	4	1
Peppers, chili, sun-dried	1 pepper	2	0	0	0	0
Peppers, jalapeno	1 pepper	4	0	0	1	0
Peppers, sweet, green	1 medium	24	0	1	6	2
Peppers, sweet, red	1 medium	31	0	1	7	2
Peppers, sweet, yellow	1 medium	32	0	1	·8	1
Persimmons	1 fruit	32	0	0	8	0
Pheasant, boneless, raw	1/2 pheasant	724	37	91	0	0
Pheasant, breast, skinless, boneless, raw	1/2 breast	242	6	44	0	0
Pheasant, leg, skinless, boneless, raw	1 leg	143	5	24	0	0
Pheasant, skinless, raw	/2 pheasant	468	13	83	0	0
Pickle relish, sweet	1 tbsp	20	0	0	5	0
Pickle, sour	1 large 4"	15	0	0	3	2
Pickle, sweet	1 large 4"	158	0	1	43	2
Pickles, dill	1 large 4"	24	0	1	6	2
Pie crust, graham cracker, baked	1 pie crust	1037	52	9	137	3
Pie, apple	1 piece	411	19	4	58	0
Pie, blueberry	1 piece	290	13	2	44	1
Pie, cherry	1 piece	325	14	3	50	1
Pie, lemon meringue	1 piece	303	10	2	53	1
Pie, pecan	1 piece	452	21	5	65	4
Pie, pumpkin	1 piece	229	10	4	30	3
Pine nuts	1 oz. (167 kernels)	191	19	4	4	1

Nutrition values for fat, protein (Prtn), carbohydrates (Cbs), and fiber (Fbr) are listed in grams per serving. Serving sizes and values are approximate.

FOOD ITEM	SERVING SIZE	CAL	FAT	PRTN	CBS	FBR
P (CONT.)						
Pineapple	1 fruit	227	1	3	60	7
Pineapple, canned	1 slice	15	0	0	4	0
Pita bread, whole wheat	1 pita	170	2	6	35	5
Pistachio nuts	1 oz. (49 kernels)	161	13	6	8	3
Pizza, cheese	1 slice (3.7 oz.)	250	10	11	29	2
Pizza, pepperoni	1 slice (3.7 oz.)	288	15	12	26	2
Plantains	1 medium	218	1	2	57	4
Plums	1 fruit	30	0	1	8	1
Plums, canned	1 plum	19	0	0	5	0
Polenta	1/2 cup	220	2	2	24	1
Pomegranates	1 fruit	105	1	2	26	1
Popcorn cakes	1 cake	38	0	1	8	0
Popcorn, air-popped	1 cup	31	0	1	6	1
Popcorn, caramel-coated	1 oz.	122	4	1	22	2
Popcorn, cheese	1 cup	58	4	1	6	1
Popcorn, oil-popped	1 cup	55	3	1	6	1
Popovers, dry mix	1 oz.	105	1	3	20	1
Poppy seed	1 tsp	15	1	1	1	0
Pork, cured, breakfast strips, cooked	3 slices	156	12	10	0	0
Pork, cured, ham, extra lean, canned	3 oz.	116	4	18	0	0
Pork, cured, ham, patties	1 patty	205	18	8	1	0
Pork, cured, ham, extra lean, cooked	3 oz.	140	7	19	0	0
Pork, cured, salt pork, raw	1 oz.	212	23	1	0	0
Pork, fresh ground, cooked	3 oz.	252	18	22	0	0
Pork, leg, rump half, cooked	3 oz.	214	12	25	0	0
Pork, leg, shank half, cooked	3 oz.	246	17	22	0	0
Pork, leg, whole, cooked	3 oz.	232	15	23	0	0
Pork, loin, blade, cooked	3 oz.	275	21	20	0	0
Pork, loin, center loin, cooked	3 oz.	199	11	22	0	0
Pork, loin, center rib, cooked	3 oz.	214	13	23	0	0
Pork, loin, sirloin, cooked	3 oz.	176	8	24	0	0
Pork, loin, tenderloin, cooked	3 oz.	147	5	24	0	0
Pork, loin, top loin, cooked	3 oz.	192	10	24	0	0
Pork, loin, whole, cooked	3 oz.	211	12	23	0	0
Pork, shoulder, arm, cooked	3 oz.	238	18	17	0	0
Pork, shoulder, blade, cooked	3 oz.	229	16	20	0	0
Pork, shoulder, whole, cooked	3 oz.	248	18	20	0	0
Pork, spareribs, cooked	3 oz.	337	26	25	0	0
Potato chips, barbecue	1 oz.	139	9	2	15	1
Potato chips, cheese	1 oz.	141	8	2	16	2
Potato chips, salted	1 oz.	152	10	2	15	1
Potato chips, sour cream & onion	1 oz.	151	10	2	15	2
Potato chips, reduced fat	1 oz.	134	6	2	19	2
Potato chips, unsalted	1 oz.	152	10	2	15	1
Potato flour	1 cup	571	1	11	133	9
Potato salad	1 cup	358	21	7	28	3
Potatoes	1 medium	164	0	4	37	5
Potatoes, baked, w/ skin	1 medium	160	0	4	37	4
Potatoes, baked, w/o skin	1 medium	143	0	3	33	3
Potatoes, mashed	1 cup	237	9	4	35	3

Nutrition values for fat, protein (Prtn), carbohydrates (Cbs), and fiber (Fbr) are
listed in grams per serving. Serving sizes and values are approximate.

FOOD ITEM	SERVING SIZE	CAL	FAT	PRTN	CBS	FBR
P (CONT.)						
Potatoes, red	1 medium	153	0	4	34	4
Potatoes, russet	1 medium	168	0	5	39	3
Potatoes, scalloped	1 cup	211	9	7	26	5
Potatoes, white	1 medium	149	0	4	34	5
Pretzels, hard, plain, salted	1 oz.	108	1	3	22	1
Prune juice	8 fl.oz.	180	0	2	43	3
Pudding, banana	1/2 cup	154	3	4	29	0
Pudding, chocolate	1/2 cup	154	3	5	28	0
Pudding, coconut cream	1/2 cup	157	3	4	28	0
Pudding, lemon	1/2 cup	157	3	4	30	0
Pudding, rice	1/2 cup	163	2	5	31	0
Pudding, tapioca	1/2 cup	154	2	4	29	0
Pudding, vanilla	1/2 cup	148	3	4	27	0
Pumpkin	1 cup	30	0	1	8	1
Pumpkin pie mix	1 cup	281	0	3	71	22
Pumpkin, canned	1 cup	83	1	3	20	7
R						
Rabbit, cooked	3 oz.	167	7	25	0	0
Radicchio	1 cup, shredded	9	0	1	2	0
Radishes	1 cup, sliced	19	0	1	4	2
Raisins	1 1/2 oz.	129	0	1	34	2
Raisins, golden	1 1/2 oz.	130	0	1	34	2
Raspberries	1 cup	64	1	2	15	8
Rhubarb	1 cup, diced	26	0	1	6	2
Rice cakes, brown rice, corn	1 cake	35	0	1	7	0
Rice cakes, brown rice, multigrain	1 cake	35	0	1	7	0
Rice cakes, brown rice, plain	1 cake	35	0	1	7	0
Rice, brown, cooked	1 cup	218	2	5	46	4
Rice, white, cooked	1 cup	242	0	4	53	1
Rice, wild	1 cup	166	1	7	35	3
Rolls, dinner	1 roll	136	3	4	23	1
Rolls, dinner, wheat	1 roll	117	3	4	20	2
Rolls, dinner, whole-wheat	1 roll	114	2	4	22	3
Rolls, french	1 roll	119	2	4	22	0
Rolls, hamburger or hotdog	1 roll	120	2	4	21	1
Rolls, hard (incl. kaiser)	1 roll	126	2	4	23	1
Rolls, pumpernickel	1 roll	119	1	5	23	2
Rosemary	1 tsp	1	0	0	0	0
Rosemary, dried	1 tsp	4	0	0	1	1
Rum, 80 proof	1 fl.oz.	64	0	0	0	0
Rutabagas	1 cup, cubed	50	0	2	11	4
Rye	1 cup	566	4	25	118	25
Rye flour, dark	1 cup	415	3	18	88	29
Rye flour, light	1 cup	374	1	9	82	15
Rye flour, medium	1 cup	361	2	10	79	15
S						
Sage, ground	1 tsp	2	0	0	0	0
Sake	1 fl.oz.	39	0	0	2	0

Nutrition values for fat, protein (Prtn), carbohydrates (Cbs), and fiber (Fbr) are listed in grams per serving. Serving sizes and values are approximate.

FOOD ITEM	SERVING SIZE	CAL	FAT	PRTN	CBS	FBR
S (CONT.)						
Salad dressing, 1000 island	1 tbsp	58	6	0	2	0
Salad dressing, bacon & tomato	1 tbsp	49	5	0	0	0
Salad dressing, blue cheese	1 tbsp	77	8	1	1	0
Salad dressing, caesar	1 tbsp	78	9	0	1	0
Salad dressing, coleslaw	1 tbsp	61	5	0	4	0
Salad dressing, french	1 tbsp	71	7	0	2	0
Salad dressing, honey dijon	1 tbsp	58	5	1	3	1
Salad dressing, italian	1 tbsp	43	4	0	2	0
Salad dressing, mayo-based	1 tbsp	57	5	0	4	0
Salad dressing, mayonnaise	1 tbsp	103	12	0	0	0
Salad dressing, peppercorn	1 tbsp	76	8	0	1	0
Salad dressing, ranch	1 tbsp	25	0	0	0	0
Salad dressing, russian	1 tbsp	76	8	0	2	0
Salad, chicken	6 oz.	420	33	45	11	2
Salad, egg	6 oz.	300	23	20	14	1
Salad, prima pasta	6 oz.	360	30	5	18	3
Salad, seafood w/ crab & shrimp	6 oz.	420	34	0	20	0
Salad, tuna	6 oz.	450	36	16	14	0
Salami, cooked, turkey	1 oz.	38	2	1	0	0
Salami, dry, pork or beef	3 slices	104	8	6	1	0
Salami, italian pork	1 oz.	119	10	6	0	0
Salsa, w/ oil	2 tbsp	40	3	0	8	0
Salsa, w/o oil	2 tbsp	15	0	0	4	0
Salt	1 tbsp	0	0	0	0	0
Sauce, alfredo	1/4 cup	120	11	15	3	2
Sauce, barbecue	1 cup	188	5	5	32	3
Sauce, cheese	1 cup	479	36	25	13	0
Sauce, cranberry	1 cup	418	0	1	108	3
Sauce, hollandaise	1 cup	62	2	2	10	0
Sauce, honey mustard	1 tbsp	30	1	0	5	0
Sauce, marinara	1 cup	185	6	5	28	1
Sauce, salsa	1 cup	70	0	4	16	4
Sauce, soy	1 tbsp	10	0	0	0	0
Sauce, steak	1 tbsp	25	0	0	6	0
Sauce, teriyaki	1 tbsp	15	0	17	2	0
Sauce, tomato chili	1 cup	284	1	7	54	16
Sauce, worcestershire	1 cup	184	0	0	54	0
Sauerkraut	1/2 cup	25	0	1	5	4
Sausage, italian pork, raw	1 link	391	35	16	1	0
Sausage, pork	1 link	85	7	4	0	0
Sausage, smoked linked, pork	1 link	265	22	15	1	0
Sausage, turkey	1 link	0	0	0	0	0
Savory, ground	1 tsp	4	0	0	1	1
Scallops	1 scallop	26	0	5	1	0
Seaweed, dried	1 oz.	50	0	0	13	0
Sesame seeds, dried	1 tbsp	52	5	2	2	1
Shallots	1 tbsp, chopped	7	0	0	2	0
Shortening	1 tbsp	113	13	0	0	0
Shrimp, mixed species, raw	1 medium piece	6	0	1	0	0
Snacks, cheese puffs or twists	1 oz.	157	10	2	15	0

Nutrition values for fat, protein (Prtn), carbohydrates (Cbs), and fiber (Fbr) are listed in grams per serving. Serving sizes and values are approximate.

FOOD ITEM	SERVING SIZE	CAL	FAT	PRTN	CBS	FBR
S (CONT.)						
Soda, club	12 fl.oz.	0	0	0	0	0
Soda, cream	12 fl.oz.	252	0	0	66	0
Soda, diet cola	12 fl.oz.	0	0	0	0	0
Soda, ginger ale	12 fl.oz.	166	0	0	43	0
Soda, lemon-lime	12 fl.oz.	196	0	0	51	0
Soda, regular, w/ caffeine	12 fl.oz.	155	0	0	40	0
Soda, regular, w/o caffeine	12 fl.oz.	207	0	0	53	0
Soda, root beer	12 fl.oz.	202	0	0	52	0
Soda, tonic water	12 fl.oz.	166	0	0	43	0
Soup, beef broth	1 cup	29	0	5	2	0
Soup, beef stroganoff	1 cup	235	11	12	22	1
Soup, beef vegetable	1 cup	82	2	3	13	1
Soup, chicken broth	1 cup	39	1	5	1	0
Soup, chicken noodle	1 cup	75	2	4	9	1
Soup, chicken vegetable	1 cup	75	3	4	9	1
Soup, chicken w/ dumplings	1 cup	96	6	6	6	1
Soup, clam chowder	1 cup	95	3	5	12	2
Soup, cream of chicken	1 cup	117	7	3	9	0
Soup, cream of mushroom	1 cup	129	9	2	9	1
Soup, cream of potato	1 cup	149	6	6	17	1
Soup, minestrone	1 cup	82	3	4	11	1
Soup, split-pea w/ham	1 cup	190	4	10	28	2
Soup, tomato	1 cup	161	6	6	22	3
Soup, vegetarian	1 cup	72	2	2	12	1
Sour cream	1 tbsp	26	2.5	0	1	0
Sour cream, fat free	1 tbsp	9	0	0	2	0
Sour cream, reduced fat	1 tbsp	22	2	1	1	0
Soy milk	1 cup	127	5	11	12	3
Soy protein isolate	1 oz.	96	1	23	2	2
Soybeans, green, cooked	1 cup	254	12	22	12	7
Soybeans, nuts, roasted	1/4 cup	194	9	17	14	3
Soyburger	1 patty	125	4	13	9	3
Spaghetti, cooked	1 cup	197	1	7	40	2
Spaghetti, spinach, cooked	1 cup	182	1	6	37	2
Spaghetti, whole-wheat, cooked	1 cup	174	1	7	37	6
Spinach	1 cup	7	0	1	1	1
Squab, boneless, raw	1 squab	585	47	37	0	0
Squab, skinless, raw	1 squab	239	13	29	0	0
Squash, summer	1 cup, sliced	18	0	1	4	1
Squash, winter	1 cup, cubed	39	0	1	10	2
Squid, mixed species, raw	1 oz.	26	0	4	1	0
Stock, beef	1 cup	31	0	5	3	0
Stock, chicken	1 cup	86	3	6	9	0
Stock, fish	1 cup	40	2	5	0	0
Strawberries	1 cup	49	1	1	12	3
Succotash	1 piece	0	0	0	0	0
Sugar, brown	1 tsp	12	0	0	3	0
Sugar, granulated	1 tsp	16	0	0	4	0
Sugar, maple	1 tsp	11	0	0	3	0
Sugar, powdered	1 tsp	10	0	0	3	0

Nutrition values for fat, protein (Prtn), carbohydrates (Cbs), and fiber (Fbr) are listed in grams per serving. Serving sizes and values are approximate.

FOOD ITEM	SERVING SIZE	CAL	FAT	PRTN	CBS	FBR
S (CONT.)						
Sunflower seeds	1 tbsp	45	10	4	2	5
Sweet potato	1 cup, cubed	114	0	2	27	4
Syrup, chocolate	1 tbsp	67	2	1	12	1
Syrup, dark corn	1 tbsp	57	0	0	16	0
Syrup, grenadine	1 tbsp	53	0	0	13	0
Syrup, light corn	1 tbsp	59	0	0	16	0
Syrup, maple	1 tbsp	52	0	0	13	0
Syrup, pancake	1 tbsp	47	0	0	12	0
T						
Taco shell, hard	1 shell	55	3	2	6	0
Tangerines	1 large	52	0	1	13	2
Tarragon, dried	1 tsp	2	0	0	0	0
Tea, instant	1 cup	2	0	0	0	0
Thyme	1 tsp	1	0	0	0	0
Thyme, dried	1 tsp	3	0	0	1	0
Tofu, firm	1/2 cup	183	11	20	5	3
Tofu, fried	1 piece	35	3	2	1	1
Tofu, soft	1/2 cup	76	5	8	2	0
Tomato juice, canned, with salt	6 fl.oz.	31	0	1	8	1
Tomato juice, canned, without salt	6 fl.oz.	30	0	1	8	1
Tomato paste, canned	1/2 cup	107	1	6	25	6
Tomato sauce, canned	1 cup	78	1	3	18	4
Tomatoes, canned, crushed	1 cup	82	1	4	19	5
Tomatoes, green	1 cup, chopped	41	0	2	9	2
Tomatoes, orange	1 cup, chopped	25	0	2	5	1
Tomatoes, red	1 cup, chopped	32	0	2	7	2
Tomatoes, sun-dried	1 cup, chopped	139	2	8	30	7
Toppings, butterscotch or caramel	2 tbsp	103	0	1	27	0
Toppings, marshmallow cream	2 tbsp	132	0	0	32	0
Toppings, nuts in syrup	2 tbsp	184	9	2	24	1
Toppings, pineapple	2 tbsp	106	0	0	28	0
Toppings, strawberry	2 tbsp	107	0	0	28	0
Tortilla chips, plain	1 oz.	142	7	2	18	2
Tortilla, corn	1 tortilla	45	1	2	9	3
Tortilla, flour	1 tortilla	160	3	18	28	3
Trail mix	1/4 cup	173	11	5	17	3
Turkey, deli sliced, white meat	1 oz.	30	1	5	1	0
Turkey, back, skinless, boneless, raw	1/2 back	180	5	31	0	0
Turkey, breast, boneless, raw	1/2 breast	541	12	103	0	0
Turkey, breast, skinless, boneless, raw	1/2 breast	433	3	96	0	0
Turkey, dark meat, boneless, raw	1/2 turkey	686	26	107	0	0
Turkey, dark meat, skinless, boneless, raw	1/2 turkey	532	13	98	0	0
Turkey, leg, boneless, raw	1 leg	412	13	70	0	0
Turkey, leg, skinless, boneless, raw	1 leg	355	8	67	0	0
Turkey, wing, boneless, raw	1 wing	204	10	27	0	0
Turkey, wing, skinless, boneless, raw	1 wing	95	1	20	0	0
Turkey, young hen, back, boneless, raw	1/2 back	650	48	52	0	0
Turkey, young hen, breast, boneless, raw	1/2 breast	1460	73	189	0	0
Turkey, young hen, dark meat, boneless, raw	1/2 turkey	1056	40	163	0	0

Nutrition values for fat, protein (Prtn), carbohydrates (Cbs), and fiber (Fbr) are listed in grams per serving. Serving sizes and values are approximate.

NUTRITION FACTS

FOOD ITEM	SERVING SIZE	CAL	FAT	PRTN	CBS	FBR
T (CONT.)						
Turkey, young hen, leg, boneless, raw	1 leg	991	49	128	0	0
Turkey, young hen, wing, boneless, raw	1 wing	470	31	45	0	0
Turkey, young tom, back, boneless, raw	1/2 back	938	58	97	0	0
Turkey, young tom, breast, boneless, raw	1/2 breast	2701	113	393	0	0
Turkey, young tom, dark meat, boneless, raw	1/2 turkey	1884	63	307	0	0
Turkey, young tom, leg, boneless, raw	1 leg	1740	78	241	0	0
Turkey, young tom, wing, boneless, raw	1 wing	654	39	71	0	0
Turnip greens	1 cup, chopped	18	0	1	4	2
Turnips	1 cup, cubed	36	0	1	8	2
V						
Vanilla extract	1 tbsp	37	0	0	2	0
Veal, breast, raw	1 oz.	59	4	5	0	0
Veal, cubed, raw	1 oz.	31	1	6	0	0
Veal, ground, raw	1 oz.	41	2	6	0	0
Veal, leg, raw	1 oz.	33	1	6	0	0
Veal, loin, raw	1 oz.	46	3	5	0	0
Veal, rib, raw	1 oz.	46	3	5	0	0
Veal, shank, raw	1 oz.	32	1	5	0	0
Veal, shoulder, arm, raw	1 oz.	37	2	6	0	0
Veal, shoulder, blade, raw	1 oz.	37	2	6	0	0
Veal, shoulder, whole, raw	1 oz.	37	2	6	0	0
Veal, sirloin, raw	1 oz.	43	2	5	0	0
Vegetable juice	8 fl.oz.	50	0	2	12	2
Vinegar	1 tbsp	2	0	0	1	0
W						
Waffles, plain	1 waffle	218	11	6	25	0
Walnuts	1 oz. (14 halves)	185	19	4	4	2
Wasabi root	1 cup, sliced	142	1	6	31	10
Water chestnuts, chinese	1/2 cup, sliced	60	0	1	15	2
Watercress	1 cup, chopped	4	0	1	0	0
Watermelon	1 cup, diced	46	0	1	12	1
Wheat bran	1 cup	125	3	9	37	25
Wheat flour, whole grain	1 cup	407	2	16	87	15
Wheat germ	1 cup	414	11	27	60	15
Whipped cream	1 cup	154	13	2	8	0
Wine, cooking	1 tsp	2	0	0	0	0
Wine, red	3-1/2 oz. glass	74	0	0	2	0
Wine, rose	3-1/2 oz. glass	73	0	0	1	0
Wine, white	3-1/2 oz. glass	70	0	0	1	0
Yam	1 cup, cubed	177	0	2	42	6
Yeast, active, dry	1 tsp	12	0	2	2	1
Yogurt, fruit, low fat	8 oz. container	118	0	6	24	0
Yogurt, fruit, whole milk	8 oz. container	250	6	9	38	0
Yogurt, plain, lowfat	8 oz. container	110	4	8	7	0
Yogurt, plain, whole milk	8 oz. container	138	7	12	11	0
Z						
Zucchini	1 medium	45	0	2	10	1

Nutrition values for fat, protein (Prtn), carbohydrates (Cbs), and fiber (Fbr) are listed in grams per serving. Serving sizes and values are approximate.